AF413751

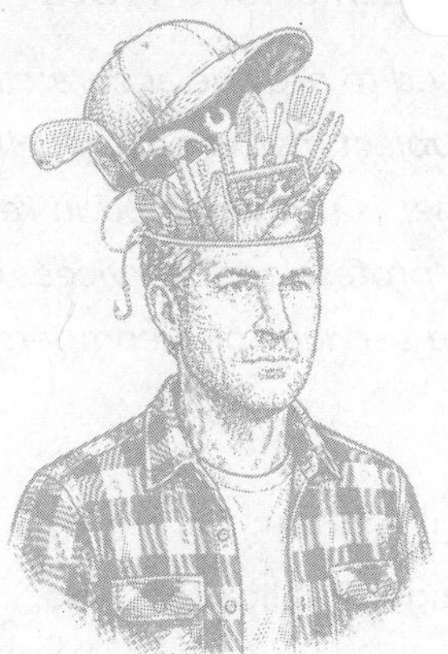

MAN THERAPY

THERAPY THE WAY A MAN DOES IT

Joe Conrad
with Matthew McKay, PhD • Stan Tatkin, PsyD
Edmund J. Bourne, PhD • Glenn R. Schiraldi, PhD
Randy J. Paterson, PhD • Michael Barnett, LPCC

New Harbinger Publications, Inc.
Man Therapy®

Publisher's Note

This publication is designed to provide accurate and authoritative information in regard to the subject matter covered. It is sold with the understanding that the publisher is not engaged in rendering psychological, financial, legal, or other professional services. If expert assistance or counseling is needed, the services of a competent professional should be sought.

NEW HARBINGER PUBLICATIONS is a registered trademark of New Harbinger Publications, Inc.

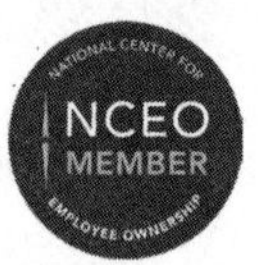

New Harbinger Publications is an employee-owned company.

Copyright © 2026 by Joe Conrad, Matthew McKay, Stan Tatkin, Edmund J. Bourne, Glenn R. Schiraldi, Randy J. Paterson, and Michael Barnett
New Harbinger Publications, Inc.
5720 Shattuck Avenue
Oakland, CA 94609
www.newharbinger.com

All Rights Reserved

Cover design by Cactus, Emma Froberg
Interior design by Tom Comitta
Acquired by Ryan Buresh
Edited by Madison Davis

Library of Congress Cataloging-in-Publication Data on file

Printed in the United States of America

28   27   26

10   9   8   7   6   5   4   3   2   1   First Printing

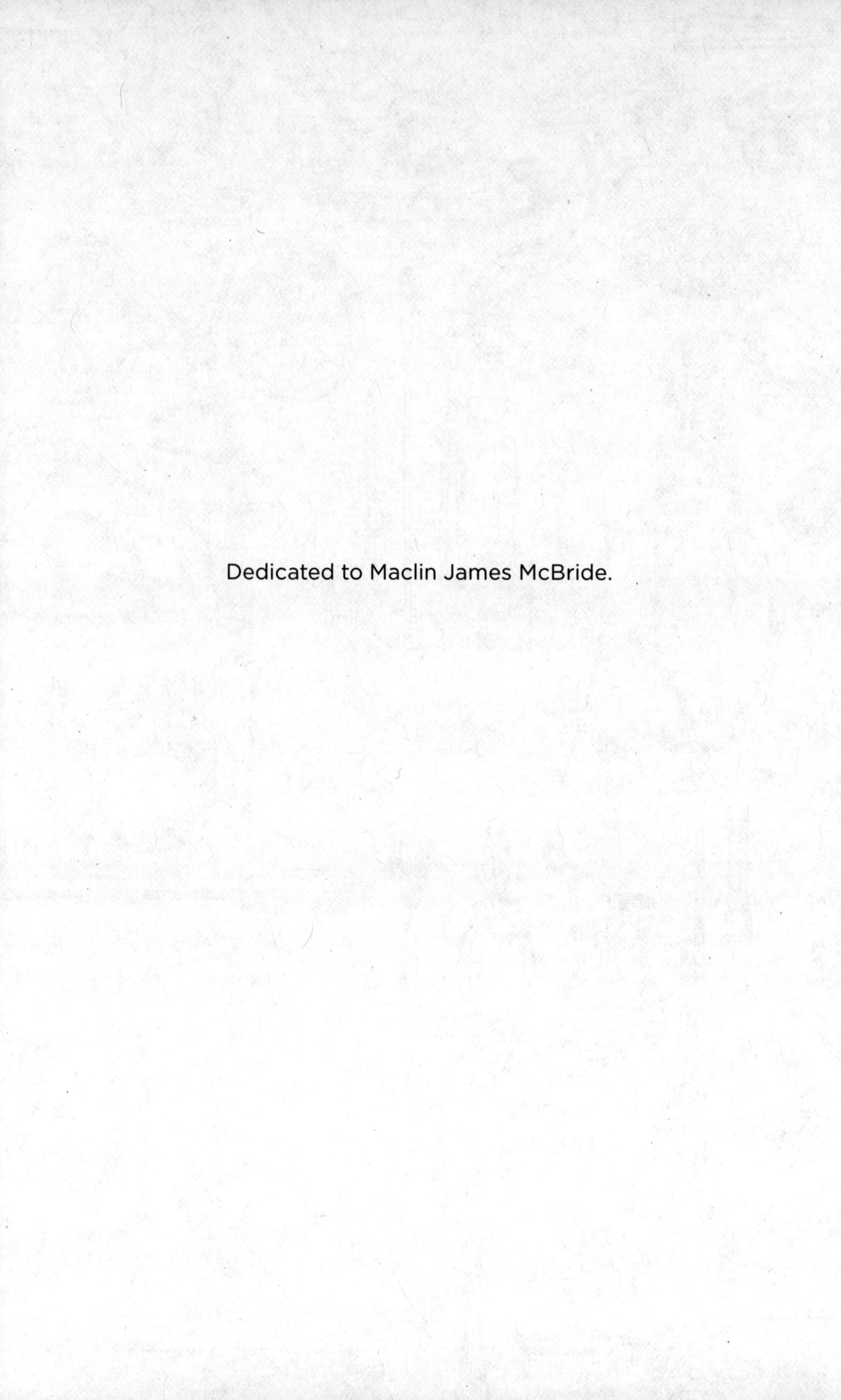
Dedicated to Maclin James McBride.

CONTENTS

FOREWORD

My business card says, "Jed Diamond, PhD: Helping men and the women who love them since 1969." That was the year I held my newborn son in my arms and made a vow that I would be a different kind of father than my father was able to be for me. I would do everything I could to create a world where men were fully healed in body, mind, and spirit.

For me, working to help men has always been personal as well as professional. When I was five years old, my father took an overdose of sleeping pills. He had become increasingly depressed because he couldn't support his family doing the work he loved and felt we all would be better off if he was gone. Fortunately, he didn't die but was instead committed to Camarillo State Mental Hospital, sixty miles north of our home in Los Angeles.

Every Sunday for over a year, I went with my uncle to visit my father, hoping that my presence would help him heal. But the kind of healthcare available to my father in 1949 was inadequate, and he continued to suffer, as do many men today. Clearly something more was needed, and it became my life work to find programs that would help men like my dad.

I first met Joe Conrad in 2019 when I came across the website Man Therapy and was introduced to Dr. Rich Mahogany, *the hardest working therapist in the world*. I was immediately impressed by how engaging the website was and even more impressed when

Joe told me that Man Therapy is an evidence-based, decades-long, multidisciplinary effort to break though stigma, improve help-seeking behavior, and reduce male suicide.

The CDC reports that men are three to four times more likely than women to die by suicide. Although suicide may be the ultimate indicator of despair, there are many other mental health issues men must deal with, including increasing levels of depression, anxiety, aggression, addictions, and loneliness.

These problems are not limited to those diagnosed by mental health professionals. They are problems throughout the world. In the past, treatment has been focused on individuals, but it is now evident that the problems are systemic and require new approaches that can be effective for engaging everyone.

The challenging issues cannot be solved simply by training more therapists or hoping that artificial intelligence will come to our rescue. Man Therapy was developed by real people, using the most up-to-date and proven methods of engagement, and has demonstrated its success helping men and their families everywhere.

The book *Man Therapy: Therapy the Way a Man Does It* is truly every man's guide to mental health. It is the guide I wish was available for my father when he lost hope and needed expert support. It is a book that can spearhead a worldwide movement to help us all reconnect with ourselves, each other, and the community of life on planet Earth. The theologian and historian Thomas Berry gave us this call to action: "We never knew enough. Nor were we sufficiently intimate with all our cousins in the great family of the earth. Nor could we listen to the various creatures of the earth, each telling its own story. The time has now come, however, when we will listen or we will die."

—Jed Diamond, author of *The Irritable Male Syndrome* and *Looking for Love in All the Wrong Places*

MENTAL HEALTH FOR ALL MEN

JOE CONRAD,
FOUNDER OF MAN THERAPY

Never forget that you are one of a kind. Never forget that if there weren't any need for you in all your uniqueness to be on this earth, you wouldn't be here in the first place. And never forget, no matter how overwhelming life's challenges and problems seem to be, that one person can make a difference in the world. In fact, it is always because of one person that all the changes that matter in the world come about. So be that one person.
—Buckminster Fuller

Consider for a moment all the amazing things men have accomplished in our brief time here on Earth. We are a curious, smart, tenacious, and passionate bunch. At the same time, men have caused most of the problems in the world when we behave with fear, greed, anger, hate, and domination. In this moment, we are still trying to determine our collective future and fate. And, as a group, men are struggling more than ever.

This book is about the personal battle that takes place inside each and every man to become the very best version of himself. We are all a work in progress. No matter our background, where we are from, what our name is, or how much money we have in the bank, we are all trying to navigate life and make the most of what we have been given. We all face challenges and struggles, and what really matters is how we meet the moment.

The truth is that everyone is on their own unique journey toward becoming the person they really want to be, regardless of their circumstances. Some adversity is actually a blessing, giving us the chance to face down challenges and overcome them. If someone faces no adversity at all, chances are they'll turn out to be an underachiever, or worse yet, a real asshole.

What doesn't kill us does indeed make us stronger. We learn a great deal about ourselves, we grow, and we're more prepared for the next time life gives us lemons. We can't change our past, what's happened to us, the genes we've inherited, or the shit that life's thrown our way, but we can control how we choose to move forward. Perhaps even more important than the challenges are the opportunities—inspiration, love, and support—waiting for us to find.

When it comes to mental health and well-being, I have discovered that the best defense is a good offense. If men can proactively deal with their shit, and more importantly, develop a growth mindset, they can unlock the power of self-determination and become more resilient in every part of their lives. Imagine the possibilities if we can reside in that place. Mental health isn't just for some guys; it's for all of us.

My Journey

By some standards, I had it easy. I am a white man who was born in 1964 in the United States, so I have been given many advantages. At the same time, I was born into a low-income, working-class family. I was the youngest of five children and the first in my family to graduate from high school and college. My life has taken twists and turns, and I have surely benefited from the support of my family, friends, church, and community.

When I was twenty-five years old and young in my professional career, I hit a dark period in my life. I was spiraling down fast, finding no joy in my work or my personal life. I found myself feeling hopeless. I was lonely, depressed, and covering it up by partying too much. A mentor of mine gave me a book that changed the course of my life: *Critical Path* by Buckminster

Fuller. Bucky, as he was affectionately known, took a vow to focus his work only on things that would benefit 100 percent of humanity. An audacious goal for sure, but one that fueled all his work and inventions. Bucky was living proof that a single person does indeed matter and an individual can have an enormous impact in the world. His life was exactly the inspiration I needed at that point in time.

The message was clear: find work that reflects my values and fuels my passion. In 1990, I started Cactus, a purpose-driven advertising agency focused on working with non-profit organizations, foundations, and brands to help bring a powerful voice to their work. Since day one, our mission has been to create sharp ideas for brands and help them thrive in harsh environments.

The Genesis of Man Therapy

In 2010, I was approached by the Colorado Office of Suicide Prevention about developing a public service campaign to address the issue of suicide among working-age men. I have always felt that creativity, innovation, and communication could solve any challenge, but I have to admit that I thought we had met our match on this one. Could a website and an ad campaign actually have a positive impact on a complex and serious issue like suicide? We decided to tackle this challenge with the same tenacious approach we always do. Our team crushed the assignment at every stage of the process—research, strategy, creative, and production—resulting in the most important work of our agency's 36-year history.

We created Man Therapy, therapy the way a man does it. Every man is somewhere on the continuum of mental health and well-being, and we wanted to appeal to all men. We built a website, ManTherapy.org, hosted by a fictional therapist, Dr. Rich Mahogany. However, Dr. Rich is not your typical therapist. He's a man's man who tells it like it is and uses a humorous, no-BS approach to show men that taking care of their mental health is the manliest thing they can do.

Man Therapy is a place where men can come to be men. No whining, just tackling the issues head on. It's about combating depression, stress, loneliness, substance abuse, anger, and other issues that are keeping men from succeeding. It's a place where men and their loved ones (wives, moms, sisters, daughters, and friends) can learn about their specific issues and develop a simple action plan for proactively addressing them with practical and effective tools. The best part is that it's all free and open 24/7/365.

Therapy comes in many forms and there are many ways to address an issue and become more resilient as a result. Formal therapy with a clinician or coach might be just what you need. However, you don't always need to see a therapist and lie on a couch to do the work. Therapy can also mean spending more quality time doing the things you love with your friends and family. You may find that the best way to deal your depression is to get out of your own head and volunteer for an organization and provide a service to others.

This collaboration with the New Harbinger team brings together Man Therapy and clinical experts who have contributed chapters on a wide range of topics. These gentlemen are a collection of some of the best minds in men's mental health. The author of each chapter delivers great information about the subject that is easy to understand while also providing simple, actionable, and useful tools you can put to work. Think of this book as a mental health field guide that you can turn to whenever you need it. You are now armed with a secret weapon on your personal journey.

We hope you learn a little about men's mental health and a little bit about yourself, and you are inspired to play offense. Onward, and most definitely upward.

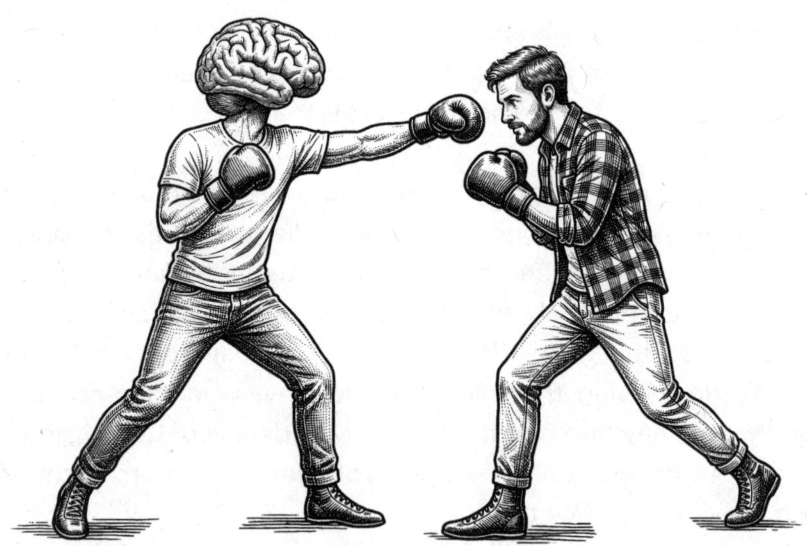

CHAPTER 1

MENTAL HEALTH

THE BEST DEFENSE IS A GOOD OFFENSE

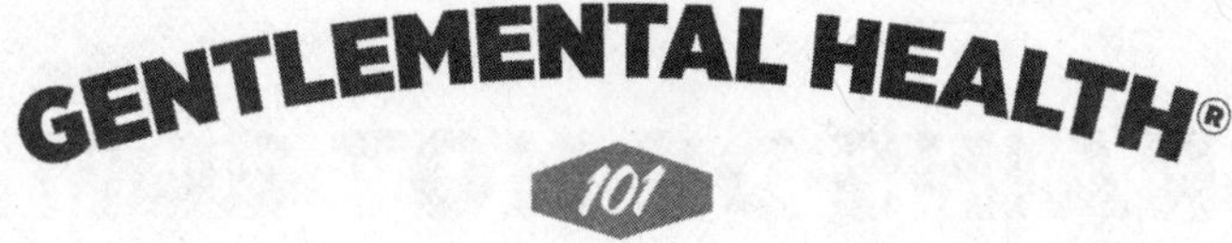

IF YOU'RE A MAN who hails from the "grin and bear it," "rub some dirt on it," or "don't you dare cry" eras, there's a good chance you've spent the bulk of your life taking the scenic route to avoid any discussions about mental health. It might be your personal belief that "mental health" is akin to terms like "gluten-free diet," "exfoliating skin scrub," or "fair-trade yoga mat." Put another way, mental health might be for others but not for you.

On the other hand, you might be a man who's a little more comfortable talking about mental health, but you can't seem to find your entry point to meaningfully engage with your own. While you can admit that things like stress, anxiety, depression, or loneliness are real, you might not have found the tools that resonate with you to address them in your life. Or you might simply not feel ready to strap on your boots and do something about it.

Wherever you are on the mental health continuum, or the specific issue you might be dealing with, we are all in the boat together. Every guy could stand to be more mentally fit and there are simple things each of us can do to get our minds in tip-top shape.

It is also mission critical to know that therapy comes in many forms. It can be an intentional conversation with a pal. It can come in the form of self-care, like getting out of your mind by stringing up a hammock and basking in the sun for a while. It might even look like extending that calloused palm of yours towards the hand of a professional to help work through something.

BRAINS DO NOT COME WITH A MANUAL

JOE CONRAD, FOUNDER OF MAN THERAPY

Unfortunately, our brains do not come with a manual. Even if they did, men probably wouldn't read it and would just try to figure it out on their own. That's why Man Therapy was created—for the self-sufficient, do-it-yourself guy who wants to jump in and fix things for himself.

Think of this book as a how-to mental health guide that tells it like it is and gives you the information and tools you need to do the work, whatever the work might be for you. For some guys it's balancing actual work and play; dealing with financial stress; feeling depressed; wrestling with the grief of losing someone close; managing a health issue; coping by consuming too much; or trying to make a relationship work. The truth is that all of us deal with all those things, and more, at one time or another.

And just when we think we have it all figured out, life can sideswipe us and leave us reeling and out of control. That's why it's important to work on your mental toughness, your resilience and your ability to successfully navigate any storm. When we are faced with a mental health challenge like anxiety, depression, anger, loneliness, addictive behavior, or even suicidal thoughts, it's important to not shy away but tackle it head on, the way a man would do it. We can celebrate all the wonderful and glorious things about men while also admitting that each of us is a beautiful and messy work in progress.

An Average Joe and Six Experts

I'm not a clinical mental health expert. I'm just a guy. A very average Joe, literally and figuratively. I come with the same amount of life experiences, challenges, dreams, habits, and baggage as anyone else. I've also had to scrap, search, learn the hard way, and discover my own path forward. Let's face it, life can be a real bastard sometimes. There are many challenges to overcome as we live and learn our way through life.

One thing men don't need is to be taught that life is hard because life itself takes care of that for us. Life is a most demanding teacher, and the goal is to learn how to survive while we strive to thrive. What's just as important though is focusing on finding joy, passion, and purpose while having fun along the way. You can't chase happiness; you need to live it every day.

My professional expertise comes from developing Man Therapy, which embraces the philosophy that the best defense is a good offense. We support men before they are in crisis by fishing upstream—helping men connect the dots and address issues early on and take charge of their mental health. We believe that mental health is not just for some of us, it's for every man. We use a straightforward, no-bullshit, and humorous approach to put the power in each of our hands to be strong and fit where it really counts: between the ears.

The following chapters provide a quick reference guide for a number of different behavioral health issues that we all might encounter somewhere along the way. I'd suggest you read the book from front to back, but please feel free to jump to a topic that is of particular interest to you. Each chapter was written by an expert in their field and covers resilience, anxiety, depression, anger, addictive behavior, and relationships. The authors are all experienced, respected professionals who are committed to helping men, and this is a unique curation of work that brings their voices together for the first time. Each chapter contains a simple explanation of a specific topic, provides sage advice, and concludes with helpful, easy-to-use tools you can put to work.

Pop the Hood:
The 20-Point Head Inspection

All of us guys are somewhere on the mental health and well-being continuum. Our position on the chart is shifting and changing all the time as we grow and wrestle with the stress and pressures of life here in the age of AI, driverless cars, and apparently aliens. Every once in a while, it's important for each of us to look in the mirror and take stock of how we're doing and acknowledge where we could use a tune-up.

Before anyone can do the work to change a behavior, the first step in the process is a deeper awareness of an issue and how it might be playing a role in your life. The second step is to gain knowledge about the topic, so you are briefed with reliable information. Armed with this knowledge, the most important step is putting it into action and doing something about it. This is how you form new and better habits.

Therapy comes in many forms and there are several things you can do to immediately feel better and make progress. There isn't a one-size-fits-all or magical solution, but you can find the remedy that works for you.

Let's give it a try. Start by taking a few minutes and do this very unique and effective breathing exercise led by Dr. Rich Mahogany, therapist in residence at **mantherapy.org**. I think it will make you feel better and you'll have a simple tool you can use whenever you feel uptight and need to get back to neutral. It might be best to do it in the privacy of your home or car, or at least out of earshot of children.

Hopefully you enjoyed that breathing exercise. I use it often and can attest to the fact that it works. Now that we're feeling relaxed, here's a fun and simple way to put your brain through its paces and see just how mentally fit you are. Go to **mantherapy.org** and take the 20-Point Head Inspection. It's fast (5 minutes), simple (20 questions), fun (you'll get a chuckle), and 100 percent free (zero strings attached)!

If you don't want to take the 20-Point Head Inspection right now, just take a few minutes to do a quick inventory on how you think you are doing when it comes to your mental health. Ask yourself about your stress levels, whether you ever get anxious, how you're sleeping, whether you feel lonely or isolated, whether you have meaningful relationships, whether you're finding enjoyment from life, whether you're leading a healthy lifestyle, whether there are some impulsive behaviors you want to address, and whether you ever have suicidal thoughts. Be honest with yourself and jot down where you are doing well and where you can be better. It'll help you understand your priorities and how you can begin tackling them.

You Can't Fix Your Mental Health with Duct Tape

A good, thick, sticky roll of duct tape can solve a lot of problems, but mental health ain't one of them. However, I believe that if you give a man the right tools, he can accomplish anything. The simple truth is that if you are honest with yourself, acknowledge the work you need to do, put together a plan, and then take action, there is nothing you can't do.

Your 20-Point Head Inspection results will come with some basic explanation of each topic and suggestions on what you can do to take action. We also created a Make A Plan feature to build on your discoveries in the Head Inspection by helping you commit to some simple steps that will point you in the right direction for your goals. The prescription for success is going to look different for each of us, and the important thing is that you find out what works best for you.

Man Therapy was created to help guys and their loved ones learn more about men's mental health, identify issues they may be wrestling with, and access a variety of free resources and tools they can put to work. There are certainly many things we can do on our own to make progress, but other times we may want to step it up and see a pro. Oftentimes, just getting more involved in our community or spending more time with family and friends will get you back on track.

The Power of Purpose and Optimism

Thank God life isn't just about wrestling demons and addressing behavioral health issues like the ones outlined in this guide. What's even more important is thinking about your hopes and dreams—taking time to reflect about what's important to you, being grateful for what you have, and imagining what could be.

Whatever energy you put out into the universe, based on your thoughts and actions, the universe answers back with connections, opportunities, and ideas. Everything in our lives and our world is connected. If you hate your job and it makes you miserable, you're going to bring that misery home. If you are drinking to excess often, it is going to poison your relationships. If you don't take care of your body, it won't take care of you. If you spend your time worrying about the future and imagining the worst, it's hard to have a hopeful outlook.

The important thing is to be aware of these connections and the important role you play in deciding what to do about it—your freedom to choose and make smart, healthy choices that serve you. Our beliefs drive our behaviors, our behaviors create our habits, and our habits create our world. What world do you want to inhabit?

While there are always going to be things that drag us down, there are just as many things that can lift us up. Helping someone in need and seeing the look on their face fills your heart. Completing something really hard like climbing a tall mountain gives you the confidence to compete. Conquering fear and not giving up makes you stronger in everything you do. Acting selflessly and being there for a friend adds meaning to life. Volunteering your time makes you feel worthy. Making progress and celebrating small victories encourages you to keep going and finish strong.

There's only one person who is responsible for you: you, yourself, and you. We all need friends and family to succeed, but at the end of the day, it is up to each of us. We all have the power to direct our thoughts and energy in whatever direction we choose. Never underestimate the power of positive thinking. And just imagine what we could accomplish if we all approach the world with tenacious optimism.

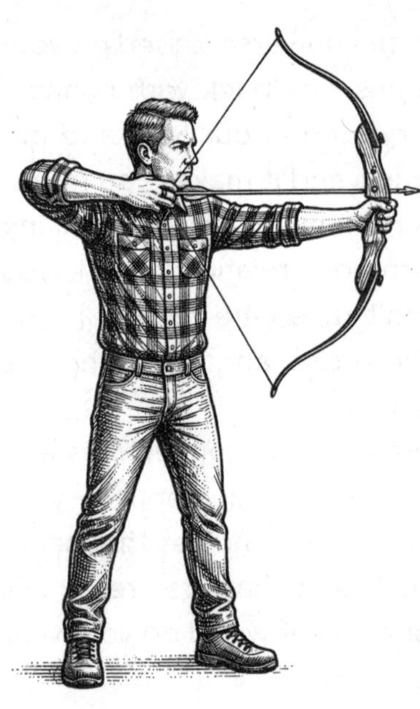

Dr. Rich's Mental Health Remedy: Learn Something New

Learning new things makes you more confident and adaptable and widens your perspective. Learning something new can kickstart you down the road to a more satisfactory life, and it can even have positive benefits on your mental and physical health. Plus, your smart-ass kid won't seem so smart anymore, will he?

Want more manly mental health tips and resources? Visit **ManTherapy.org**.

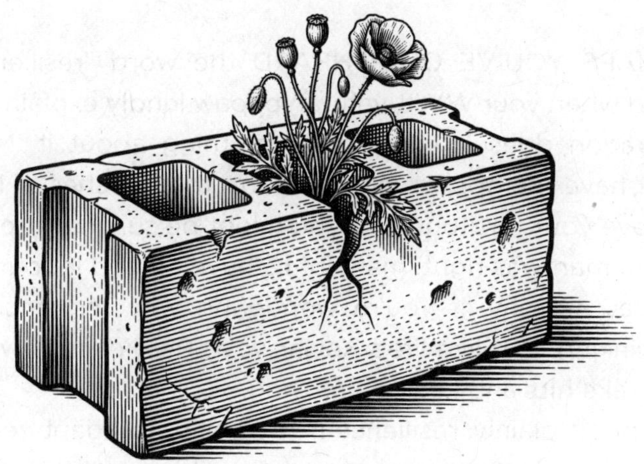

CHAPTER 2

RESILIENCE

PEACE THROUGH STRENGTH

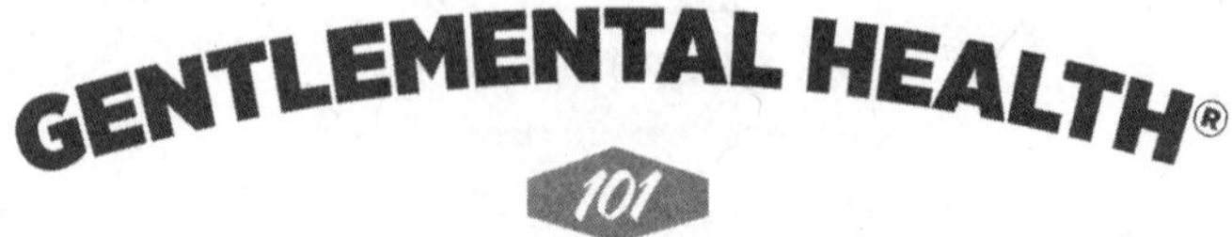

PERHAPS YOU'VE ONLY HEARD the word "resilience" mentioned when your WWII-veteran papaw kindly explains that your generation doesn't know the first thing about it. Maybe you didn't have the opportunity to storm the beaches of Normandy to prove your fortitude, but you might be surprised to learn that the old man was right: many of us have indeed let our resilience muscles atrophy. If you're wondering why resilience matters, try thinking of it like life's Kevlar vest. Resilience is what allows us to take hits and keep on moving.

To put it plainly, resilience is the ability to adapt, recover, and grow through stress, loss, and adversity. It isn't the absence of struggle; it's the ability to effectively deal with the struggles you face. While we all possess the inherent traits to develop mental fortitude, resilience, like any muscle, takes care and attention to build up over time. Knowing that every man faces a multitude of challenges, it is important to stock your toolbelt with strategies that ensure you're equipped to roll with the punches.

Now, if you're worried that you've heard this "cowboy up" bit before, it's helpful to remember that resilience is not simply a matter of toughening up. Resilience is a flexible strength that allows even the manliest of men to acknowledge their pain, adjust to it, and take action, as opposed to burying feelings and white-knuckling it down life's highway.

Ultimately, resilience combats the urge to withdraw and suppress, and taps into a man's desire to solve problems, adapt to tough environments, build community, and find a path forward. Strategies for cultivating resilience can range from adjusting behavior patterns and routines, to adapting a growth mindset (for example, reframing "I can handle this alone" to "I should get help and learn from this"), to setting healthy boundaries, to accepting things as they are, to finding resiliency role models, and more.

If you're looking for a well-balanced resilience diet, try equal parts mindset, support network, coping skills, and flexibility. And remember, resilience in one area of your life often spills over into other areas, helping you tackle the expected and unexpected challenges thrown your way.

Now, let's hear from the expert, Glenn Schiraldi, on the importance of developing resilience and effective strategies to harness it in your life.

BUILDING RESILIENCE

GLENN R. SCHIRALDI, PHD

Resilience comprises those inner strengths of mind and character—both inborn and developed—that enable one to respond well to adversity, including the capacities to:

- prevent stress-related conditions, such as depression or anxiety, or their recurrence;

- recover faster and more completely from stress and stress-related conditions; and

- optimize mental fitness and functioning in the various areas of life.

As this definition suggests, resilience is standard issue, meaning that we all already possess the strengths of mind and character in embryo—like seeds that can be grown. You wouldn't have survived this long if you completely lacked resilience. And you have the capacity to greatly expand your resilience.

Responding *well* to adversity suggests that we adapt calmly and capably to changing circumstances, drawing upon available strengths—be they mental, spiritual, emotional, physical, finan-cial, or social (for example, mentors, family, or friends).

Resilience is a process and a staircase. You might be on step four of the staircase, and I might be on step one, but we can both keep moving up the staircase so that our resilience levels will hopefully exceed the rising tide of stress. You can enlarge your capacity for resilience by practicing resilience skills. As we build resilience, health and functioning typically improve.

Why Is Resilience So Important?

First, resilience counters the *psychological* problems that trouble so many of us. Approximately 50 percent of American adults (Kessler et al. 1994, 2005) will experience a stress-related condi-tion, and prevalence rates for these conditions are increasing globally. Much of this suffering is needless. Resilience can largely prevent these conditions from developing or recurring. Should these conditions occur, resilience can reduce symptom severity and facilitate recovery.

Second, resilience counters many *medical* and *functional* prob-lems. The emotional toll of stress-related conditions is bad enough. However, the mind and body are connected. So excessive, unre-solved emotional stress makes us more vulnerable to a wide range of medical diseases, earlier death, and impaired functioning at work, home, and play.

Third, resilience is about mastery and growth. Resilience does more than fight problems; it promotes optimal well-being. Resilience helps us thrive mentally, emotionally, physically, socially, and spiri-tually—and function at our best, especially during difficult times. With resilience, we tend to be calmer, more productive, and enjoy life more. Conversely, those who lack resilience tend to have higher rates of absenteeism and of prematurely leaving their careers.

While everyone is resilient to some degree, no one is perfectly resilient, or resilient in all circumstances. Resilience does not mean invulnerability, because anyone can be overwhelmed when circumstances are severe enough. Rather, resilience is about generally working, playing, loving, and expecting well (Werner 1992) and functioning at our best possible level in any given situation. As the legendary coach John Wooden taught his highly successful basketball players, success is doing *your* personal best; sometimes the other team will simply be better on a given day.

Prepping Yourself for Hard Things

Resilience starts with the brain. Most people do not fully appreciate how the physical conditioning of the brain profoundly affects mental health and functioning. The resilient brain functions at optimal efficiency. It learns, remembers, sizes up problems, follows instructions, plans, executes decisions, and regulates moods. And it does all this relatively quickly, even under duress. The resilient brain also resists and reverses cognitive decline and brain cell death.

REGULAR EXERCISE

Many studies document the ways exercise, particularly aerobic exercise, benefit mood and brain function. Exercisers have sharper brains at all ages. Exercise produces master molecules in the brain that normally decrease with stress and aging. These master molecules increase blood flow to the brain, strengthen and grow neurons, increase antioxidants, and prime neurons to learn new coping skills. Exercise reduces tension, anxiety, and depression, often as well as prescribed medications do and without side effects, while improving sleep and increasing energy. When started gradually and done in moderation, regular exercise usually strengthens joints and reduces pain. It has been found to even reduce PTSD symptoms.

BRAIN-HEALTHY NUTRITION

A growing number of studies have shown that a Mediterranean-style diet greatly promotes longevity, brain health, and sharper brain function. This type of diet emphasizes fruits and vegetables (fresh or frozen), fish, whole grains, nuts and seeds, beans and peas, and olive oil; moderate amounts of poultry, eggs, and low-fat dairy; and minimal red and processed meats (beef, lamb, pork, hot dogs, sausage, salami, and other lunch meats), butter, stick margarine, cheese, pastries and sweets, and fried or fast food. Here are some other helpful nutrition guidelines.

Maximize the intake of brain-friendly antioxidants. These protect neurons from damage caused by stress and aging. Antioxidants are found in colorful fruits and vegetables—fresh or frozen.

Aim to eat at least two to three servings of fish per week, totaling at least eight ounces. The omega-3 fatty acids in fish are critical components of the brain's neurons. These fatty acids improve brain health and function, while reducing depression and possibly even stress. Restrict the amount of fried fish you consume, since frying adds unhealthy fats and cancels the benefits.

Choose good carbohydrates. The brain functions best with a steady supply of blood sugar. Plant foods, as nature packages them, contain fiber, which slows the absorption of sugars and provides that steady supply of sugar. So emphasize whole grains and fresh or frozen plant foods, which will also help you stay lean.

Choose good fats. Replace saturated fats and the trans fats found in processed and fast foods—think of a hamburger on a bun made from refined white flour—with healthy fats found in plant foods. Healthy fats include olive oil, avocados, and nuts.

Hydrate. Neurons are mostly water. Mood and mental functioning can be impaired by consuming too little liquid. Assuming normal eating, you will likely need to drink nine to sixteen cups of liquid a day to properly hydrate—or even more if you are large or active, even in cooler conditions. Drink throughout the day.

Spread out protein intake throughout the day. Start with a good breakfast, which sharpens the brain, promotes a sense of fullness throughout the day, and promotes leanness. Protein can come from low- or no-fat unsweetened yogurt, egg whites, poultry, seafood, beans, nuts, peanut butter, or protein powder.

Eat enough, but not too much. The combination of consuming needed nutrients but not overeating appears to help neurons rest and regenerate.

Minimize added salt and sugar.

SLEEP

Can you remember that last time you got a good night's sleep and the world seemed brighter and people more pleasant? Sleep energizes and refreshes the brain. A good night's sleep also reduces oxidative stress and helps clear toxins from the brain. Yet most of us do not fully appreciate how even a little sleep deprivation significantly impairs mental health and performance. Most adults require between 7 and 8¼ hours of sleep per night to feel and function their best. Less than that amount worsens mood and functioning.

Three principles of good sleep: There are three principles to be aware of that can help you get good sleep: amount, regularity, and quality. In terms of amount, strive for seven to eight hours of sleep per night, or even a little more. Sufficient sleep usually helps people accomplish more during the next day. Regarding regularity, try to go to bed and arise at the same time, even on weekends. Consistency helps the brain regulate sleep cycles and improve sleep. Should you need to change your schedule, try to shift the time you go to bed by less than one hour from one night to the next. Lastly, the quality of your sleep is important.

MINIMIZE SUBSTANCE USE

Smoking greatly increases the risk of depression, anxiety, and panic attacks. It also impairs memory and increases the risk of dementia. Like tobacco, marijuana decreases blood flow to the brain and impairs memory.

Alcohol intake is inversely correlated with resilience. It may even shrink the brain when taken regularly in small amounts described as "mild" or "moderate" drinking.

Excessive caffeine can interfere with brain function by restricting blood flow to the brain, and it can cause insomnia, anxiety, and excess arousal. Up to four hundred milligrams of caffeine a day—about the amount in four cups of coffee—appears to be safe for most healthy adults. This amount can easily be exceeded by drinking energy drinks, caffeinated sodas, or more than four cups of coffee.

MAKE YOUR PLAN FOR A RESILIENT BRAIN

Many people have reported that making and sticking to an exercise, nutrition, and eating plan were among the most helpful aspects of resilience training. Make a health plan that you can maintain as you work through this book and beyond. Describe your plan on a piece of paper.

Exercise: Aim to get at least 150 minutes of aerobic exercise (such as brisk walking or cycling all or most days) per week. You might also add strength and flexibility training to further sharpen the brain.

Sleep: I'll get _____ hours of sleep per night (a little more than I think I need), going to bed at _____ and getting up at _____.

Nutrition: Eat at least three times per day, selecting brain-healthy choices.

Track your progress over a fourteen-day period; then make helpful adjustments and continue to follow your plan as you move through your life. Some people find it helpful to post the plan on the fridge or someplace they will see it often.

Handling Difficult Life Transitions

Present difficulties often stir up painful emotions, which often stir up similar emotions and unresolved memories from the past. Pain from the past, in turn, can fuel worries about the future. It's reassuring to realize that distressing emotions are common to everyone, and that they usually make sense when we consider one's life experience. Perhaps you can take a moment to consider your own life experience. Have you ever experienced any of the following?

- Everyday strains (overwhelming time demands, critical leaders or family members, financial concerns, pressures to excel, ongoing conflict with family or coworkers)

- Serious illness or injury in yourself or those you care for

- Rejection, betrayal

- Humiliation, criticism, feeling inadequate

- Losing your job

- Loss (death of a loved one or friend, end of a relationship, loss of income)

- Infidelity

- Divorce (your own or that of your parents)

- Failure

- Trauma (experiencing, witnessing, or sometimes even learning about overwhelming events such as combat, terrorism, natural disasters, riots, crime, traffic accidents, domestic violence, physical or emotional abuse, or sexual trauma; rape, abuse, and molestation are particularly distressing)

Pause to reflect, again without judging. Do any of these events stir up emotions that seem strong or unsettled? Might there be connections between your everyday emotions and past experiences?

If unresolved, emotional upheaval from the past can keep present emotions highly charged, disrupting mood, physical health, and functioning. Most adults have experienced at least one such adversity. The more childhood adversities one has experienced, the more likely one is to experience psychological, medical, and functional problems (Felitti 2002). We also know that nearly every kind of trauma, particularly if it has not been resolved, is linked to increases in diverse medical conditions, ranging from the flu to even heart attacks and cancer (Prigerson et al. 1997).

This understanding underscores the importance of processing and settling past emotional wounds—the sooner the better. Fortunately, there are many ways to do this.

AVOIDING EMOTIONS USUALLY DOESN'T HELP

It is *natural* to want to avoid painful emotions, memories, or situations. However, the problem with avoidance is that nothing changes, and sometimes the very things we do to avoid pain create their own set of problems. The following lists ways that people avoid. Do any of these describe your typical response to stress? Check those that apply.

- I don't think about troubling thoughts, emotions, situations, or memories and thus do little to modify them.

- I deny anything is wrong, or I minimize the pain. ("It doesn't really bother me. It used to, but now it doesn't.")

- I numb my emotions. (When we numb negative emotions, we also numb positive emotions.)

- I dwell on physical pain or symptoms to avoid emotional pain.

- I withdraw from people, places, or situations that are distressing.

- I keep feelings to myself and don't tell others what is going on inside.

- I wish I could erase painful memories. (This is not possible, and trying to do so only creates tension.)

- I try to escape or block out negative emotions with:
  - Drugs
  - Painkillers
  - Excessive humor
  - Workaholism

- Intellectualizing (habitually thinking, complaining, worrying, or being stuck on "why" questions while not acknowledging underlying emotions and trying to resolve them)
- Overconfidence or overachieving (an attempt to compensate)
- Compulsive gambling, shopping, sex, or other addictions

What do you notice? Do you see any patterns? Might avoidance be working for or against you? Avoidance takes a lot of energy and is exhausting. It keeps us stuck emotionally and prevents us from enjoying many of life's satisfactions. Please note that habitual avoidance is not the same as healthy, temporary distractions, such as wholesome recreational activities or vacations. We are talking about habitual avoidance patterns like those listed above that do not change our *response* to pain. These patterns offer short-term benefits, and people engage in them because they haven't yet learned a better response to pain. Fortunately, there is a better strategy.

ACTIVITY
Sitting with Distressing Emotions

Meditation teaches us to be calm and nonreactive in the presence of whatever emotions arise, be they pleasant or unpleasant. Rather than trying to fight or suppress pain, we turn gently toward pain with kind awareness—relaxing and softening into it. Softening our response changes the way we experience pain. It is recommended that you practice this meditation for thirty minutes or more each day for at least a week.

Assume the meditator's posture, sitting comfortably erect, with feet flat on the floor and hands resting comfortably in the lap. The spine is straight like a stack of golden coins. The upper body is relaxed but comfortably erect, sitting in graceful dignity like a majestic mountain. Allow your eyes to close. Let your breathing help you to settle into your peaceful wisdom mind.

Remember especially the attitudes of compassion, acceptance, good humor, and vastness. Remember that you are already whole. Use the beginner's mind as you explore a new way to experience feelings.

Be aware of your breathing. For several minutes let your belly be soft and relaxed, paying attention to its rise and fall as you breathe in and out. Notice the movements and sensations in the abdomen, chest, nose, throat, and rib cage.

Be aware of any feeling in your body, any sensation as it comes and goes, without judging or trying to change it. Just notice what you sense, without judgments, such as *I don't like discomfort*. Simply notice sensations with kind acceptance and allowance. Sometimes sensations change when we bring kind awareness to them—they come and go. Nevertheless, just watch what happens without trying to make something happen. When you are ready, take a more intentional in-breath, breathe out, and then let attention dissolve from that area as you bring attention to another region of your body, such as your chest. Notice what you sense in the region around your chest. If there is any discomfort or anxiety, simply notice that. Breathe into that area.

Whenever you find your mind wandering, congratulate yourself for noticing this. This is just what the ordinary mind does. Remember that thoughts are just thoughts and not who you are, and bring your awareness gently back to breathing and sensing your body.

And now recall a difficult situation, perhaps involving work or a relationship, and the feelings that arise, such as unworthiness, inadequacy, sadness, or worry about the future. Make a space for this situation. Give deep attention to these feelings. Whatever you are feeling is all right. Greet these feelings cordially, as you would greet an old friend.

Notice where in the body you feel the feelings. It could be your stomach, chest, or throat, for example. Let yourself feel the feelings completely, with full acceptance. Don't think *I'll tighten up and let these feelings in for a minute in order to get rid of them.* This is not full acceptance. Rather, create a space that allows you to completely accept the feelings.

Breathe into that region of the body with great compassion. Follow your breath all the way down through the nose, throat, lungs, and then to the part of the body where you sense the distressing emotion or emotions. Then follow the breath out of your body, until you find yourself settling. Don't try to change or push the discomfort away. Don't brace yourself against or struggle with it. Just embrace it without judging it—with real acceptance, deep attention, peace, and goodwill and kind feelings toward all people.

Remember that you are vast enough to embrace the pain with kindness. If you find it helpful, think of loved ones who remind you of loving-kindness—and let that loving-kindness penetrate your awareness as you remember that difficult situation. Simply notice what happens to the feelings without trying to change them.

When you are ready, take a deeper breath into that area of the body, and as you exhale, widen your focus to your body as a whole. Pay attention to your whole body's breathing, being aware of the wholeness and the vast, unlimited compassion of the wisdom mind that will hold any pain that comes and goes. Expand your attention to the sounds you are hearing, just bringing them into awareness without commenting or judging. Simply listen with a half-smile. Feel the air against your body; sense your whole body breathing. Notice all that you are aware of with a soft and open heart.

To conclude, say the following intentions silently to yourself: "May I remember loving-kindness. May I be happy. May I be whole."

Be mindful of what you are now experiencing. With curiosity and good humor, just notice how your body feels. What emotions are you feeling? Is there calmness, peace, or a feeling of being settled? Are you upset? Whatever you feel, it's okay. Just let yourself be aware.

The Active Coper

Mindfulness training teaches us that the active coper turns *toward* problems, rather than away from them. This increases the likelihood of finding an appropriate response. People with an active stance toward life do the following. In order to raise your self-awareness, place a check next to those that describe you. Active copers:

Are proactive doers and problem solvers. That is, they are engaged in life. They anticipate and prepare for difficulties, rather than waiting for crises to strike. They appraise situations and take reasonable action, applying (and in some cases learning) needed skills.

Are adventurous. This means they are disposed to cope with the new and unknown.

Are curious. Curious people don't get down when they feel stress but approach problems with pleasant and engaged interest.

Acknowledge that a problem exists. They think about it, generate and weigh alternative solutions, make and follow a plan of action, and have a backup plan.

Are conscientious. That is, they are determined to build a better life and improve. So they work hard, persist, and make use of needed resources (for example, they seek out confidants, uplifting relationships, or needed information and help).

Are disciplined. They organize—creating structure, order, and routine. They follow through with their plans. They train themselves to forgo immediate pleasures and destructive shortcuts in the pursuit of a long-term goal. They act despite difficulties, fears, and risks.

Keep dreams and make goals. These goals are guided by internal core values, not the dictates of others.

Make decisions without perfect knowledge (which we never have). They allow themselves the freedom to take decisive action, take reasonable risks, make mistakes, and even fail. They realistically recognize personal and situational limitations (that is, what can and can't be done).

Recognize emotional needs and the need for emotional survival skills. They may block out emotions in order to function during a crisis, but then they address them as soon as it is appropriate so that the emotions don't continue to trouble them.

Are not impulsive. They think their actions through as much as possible before acting. They think about what they are doing and do not take unreasonable risks.

Maintain focus. They continuously ask, "What's the most important thing to do right now to get me closer to my goal?"

In *I Love a Fire Fighter*, Dr. Ellen Kirschman (2004) describes an active stance toward troubling emotions, as well as a model for dealing with them: act during the crisis, then acknowledge and process distressing feelings. She describes a water rescue training in a storm, during which a boat capsized. Afterward, one emotionally courageous firefighter said to his assembled comrades, "I don't know about you guys but I thought I was going to die out there today and I doubt I'm the only one who felt that way" (180). One by one crewmembers opened up, expressing their fears of never seeing family again and of going out on the water again, anger at firefighters' dying so young, and sadness for an incomplete life. Acknowledging these feelings brought this team together. The next day everyone went out again on the water to train. Until they had talked, each person felt isolated. Realizing that they were all in the same boat emotionally actually helped them move past their feelings and prepare for their training. Conversely, many highly trained and capable emergency service providers are engaged at work in their physical tasks, but then disengage from their feelings when they come home, shutting down or burying their emotions.

HOW TO CULTIVATE ACTIVE COPING

We can choose our response to adversity, whether that's to relax into a given situation and act to the best of our ability (which is all anyone can ever do), or to try to escape it. We can:

Acknowledge a problem. Whether it is family disharmony or the threat of terrorism, develop an action plan and rehearse it, despite resistance from other people. Recall that Rick Rescorla anticipated the terrorist attack on the World Trade Center, developed an action plan of escape, and drilled his people repeatedly until they were able to successfully execute the plan under pressure—despite the complaints of those who lacked his vision.

Drop the battle with distressing thoughts, memories, emotions, images, and sensations. Instead of fighting them, avoiding them, or giving into them in passive resignation, we can actively accept them—turning toward them and inviting them in with compassionate acceptance, as mindfulness training directs. At first we do this in quiet and calm moments. Eventually, we can kindly accept the full range of emotions even in crises and respond to them calmly so that we can perform optimally. For example, we might acknowledge fear calmly and without judgment, and then act effectively. Otherwise, fear can immobilize us or lead to frenzied reactions.

Reframe problems as challenges. Approach challenges with optimism, which is the attitude that leads to active coping. Likewise, think about our purposes in life—our reasons to survive—as these motivate us to act productively.

Use calming skills to help us see options clearly, and then act. Rehearse calming skills repeatedly under both calm and real-life training conditions.

Filling Up Your Cup with More than Beer

You've learned many skills to strengthen your brain, regulate stress, and manage strong, distressing emotions. You are now prepared for an extremely important part of resilience training: growing happiness. As you'll see, what makes us happier helps us "spiral upward," or flourish, and become more resilient overall.

The broaden and build theory of leading positive psychology researcher Dr. Barbara Fredrickson (2009) explains how happiness helps us flourish. Pleasant emotions expand our view of adversity, helping us see a broader range of coping options. They also motivate us to act on new coping options. Applying a broader range of coping options builds new neural pathways in the brain—and a larger coping repertoire for future adversity. The mechanism may be related to brain biochemistry. Pleasant emotions cause the brain to secrete neurotransmitters such as dopamine and opioids. These chemicals foster one's tendency to approach and solve problems (rather than avoid them) and reinforce or reward coping efforts with more positive feelings. An upward spiral is created whereby positive emotions lead to more effective coping, which increases satisfaction levels and the openness to tackle more challenges. Thus, happiness researcher Sonja Lyubomirsky (2007) has concluded that feeling happier makes people more productive, likable, energetic, healthy, friendly, helpful, resilient, and creative.

CAN WE BE HAPPY ALL THE TIME?

In an imperfect world, perpetual happiness is an unrealistic expectation. Most would find constant euphoria boring and shallow. Constant happiness does not favor optimal functioning. Down times can send us back to the drawing board to become wiser, stronger, and more compassionate. Strive for greater happiness, but not perfect happiness. The pursuit of perfect or constant happiness can be exhausting and disappointing.

Happy people do experience distress. For example, it is perfectly normal to feel grief and guilt at times. However, happy people spend less time feeling negative emotions, and when they do they know how to bounce back.

HOW MUCH HAPPINESS IS BEST?

There are times when being too attached to happiness, and not being open to all emotions, can work against us. For example, a person who is overly attached to happiness might minimize medical symptoms or ignore a doctor's advice. However, Dr. Fredrickson (2009) has found that people generally flourish by increasing the ratio of positive emotions to negative emotions they experience. She found that a positivity ratio of at least three to one builds resilience over time. That is, for every unpleasant emotion you experience, you need to experience at least three positive emotions to offset it. Most people fall below that ratio. The ratio can be increased by either reducing gratuitous negativity or increasing the positives. Eliminating cognitive distortions is an example of reducing negativity. Being open to the simple beauties around us is an example of increasing the positives.

ACTIVITY
Filling Your Cup

Each night, list up to five things you are grateful for from the previous twenty-four hours. Briefly describe each—how it makes you feel, what it means to you, and what the goodness is that made the moment turn out well (for example, the goodness of nature, others, God, or yourself). The point is to savor the feelings as you reminisce, so don't be overly analytical, intellectual, or emotionally detached. Do this for about five minutes each night over a two-week period. Alternatively, pick one night a week and write about five things you are thankful for from the past week. Keep this up for six to ten weeks or longer. Some find that spreading out the journal writing keeps the process fresher. Experiment to find a frequency that works best for you.

Write about anything that makes you happier or enriches your life, big or small.

Accomplishments or successes (yours and others')

A scene in nature, beautiful surroundings

Something you learned

Uplifting principles

Things in progress (goals, opportunities, possibilities to anticipate)

Tender mercies (kindnesses provided by others, nature, or Providence)

Pride in surviving, personal strengths

To strengthen your writing experience, you might add photos, letters, quotations, or other mementos to your journal. You might practice heart coherence—experiencing gratitude for a memory at the heart level. During the day, be on the hunt or alert for things you are grateful for, such as sounds in nature, the aroma of food, or a child's innocent facial expression.

EXPRESS GRATITUDE TO OTHERS FREQUENTLY

To waitresses, protectors, or people working in businesses, say, "Thanks for your help." Be genuine and specific ("I really appreciated the way you…"). If service is especially good, tell the supervisor. This makes three people feel good: the appreciated worker, the supervisor, and yourself.

Teachers might especially appreciate this story. Mark Medoff (1986), the playwright and screenwriter of *Children of a Lesser God*, returned to his school. He introduced himself to a favorite teacher as a student of hers from many years before. She cocked her head, hoping the angle might jog her memory. He wanted to deliver a perfectly worded message. Instead, all he could say was, "I wanted you to know you were important to me." There in the hallway, this lovely, dignified lady began to weep. She encircled him in her arms and whispered, "Thank you!" before disappearing back into her classroom. Gratitude lifted the spirits of two people that day. The ripple effect undoubtedly benefited the students that day, as well. Remember to thank loved ones often. It strengthens bonds.

SHARE GRATITUDE EXPERIENCES WITH LOVED ONES AT THE END OF THE DAY

It is pleasant to hear about what went well and what has been working. By making time together more enjoyable, this process can strengthen relationships. This is an enjoyable way to tuck children into bed, which also helps them to cultivate the habit of gratitude. You might also ask children how they might thank someone for giving them a gift.

ACTIVITY
Strengthening Optimistic Beliefs

Optimistic beliefs can be reinforced in many ways.

Read books that reveal the optimistic thinking of resilient survivors. Excellent examples are the autobiographies of Arthur Ashe (the tennis star who contracted AIDS through a blood transfusion) and WWII survivors Viktor Frankl and Irene Opdyke.

Collect and ponder reflections regarding optimism.

It is a peculiarity of man that he can only live by looking to the future...and this is his salvation in the most difficult moments of his existence, although he sometimes has to force his mind to the task. **—Viktor Frankl**

Freedom is nothing else but a chance to be better, whereas enslavement is a certainty of the worst. **—Albert Camus**

The optimist sees opportunity in every danger; the pessimist sees danger in every opportunity. **—Winston Churchill**

We are troubled on every side, yet not distressed; we are perplexed, but not in despair. **—2 Corinthians 4:8**

ACTIVITY
How to Grow Moral Strength

Decide in advance to live morally, and then do so. The best time to make decisions about what you will or will not do is before adversity strikes. Once a moral course has been predetermined, it is considerably easier to act with integrity when you're under duress, tired, or tempted.

Have a system for righting, and making peace with, wrongs that you will inevitably make because you are human. Starting anew, bouncing back from mistakes or bad choices, is a critical part of resilience. We might call this moral resilience. In many cultures, religions, and recovery groups, these are the steps:

Admit the wrong. We can't change what we deny.

Make amends when possible. This is the compassionate thing to do as it is healing for the offended party and ourselves. Sometimes a sincere apology is all that can be given.

Acknowledge mitigating circumstances (for example, "I was inexperienced," "I made a decision under pressure," or "I didn't have all the facts"). This is not making excuses, just increasing understanding. I'll always remember my West Point company mate, Doug Madigan, with appreciation. At a class reunion, I shared with him my biggest regret from West Point. Two of my roommates during plebe year flunked out, and I wondered whether, if I had been a better friend, they might have made it. Doug, who was friendly with both of the roommates, said with genuine concern, "What did we know when we were eighteen?" Somehow, that made me feel better. In a more general sense, what do we know when we are thirty or fifty years old? We are all still learning and trying to get the hang of living well.

Acknowledge your right to pick yourself up after falling. Worthwhile people don't lose their worth because of imperfections, nor do they forfeit their right to keep trying to improve.

Reconcile with a higher power. For example, ask for forgiveness, allowing God to take the pain and trusting that forgiveness will come.

Forgive yourself. Some become depressed, dispirited, and even suicidal because of an act or a pattern of transgression. They might conclude they are beyond redemption or can never again be good enough after doing that. Following the suggestion of Follette and Pistorello (2007), you might ask yourself, "Have I stopped valuing [honesty, kindness, virtue] just because I strayed from the path, or got turned around once, twice, or even for several years?"

Commit to a better course of action, resolving not to repeat the mistake. Have the wisdom to change course, then do your earnest best. That's all we would ask of our children. And if you then stumble, try again. Growing moral strength is a lifelong process.

ACTIVITY
Finding Meaning in Adversity

Identify a current problem, such as conflict, the end of a relationship, having too much to do, a troubled family member, a move, major life changes, the illness or death of a loved one, or your own illness. Take time to ponder and then respond to these questions in writing.

How could this problem change your life in a positive way?

Which of your strengths does this situation require?

Has anything good come out of dealing with this problem so far?

How might you benefit from this situation in the long term?

How might this situation prepare you for adversity in the future?

How might others benefit in the long term as a result of this situation or the things you've suffered?

What might you learn from this experience?

What can you still feel good about?

What in life is still important to you despite this experience?

Additional questions to consider:

What inner strengths have kept you from suffering more than you might have?

What has kept you going?

What is life still expecting of you?

What keeps you from quitting?

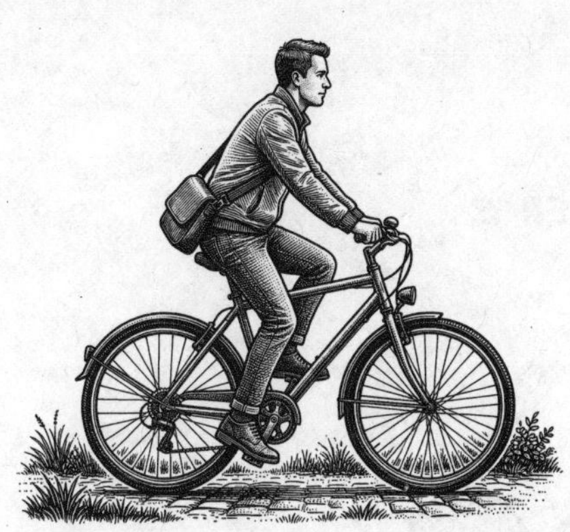

Dr. Rich's Resilience Remedy: Cycling

Cycling might be a pain in the nuts, but it's a great way to get outside and get the blood pumping. It also proves that, no matter how steep, with a little gristle and gumption, a man can charge up any hill. Next time you're feeling down, stressed, or pissed, pedal around for an hour. You just might feel yourself feeling better.

Want more manly tips on Resilience? Explore the Gentlemental Health card on **ManTherapy.org**.

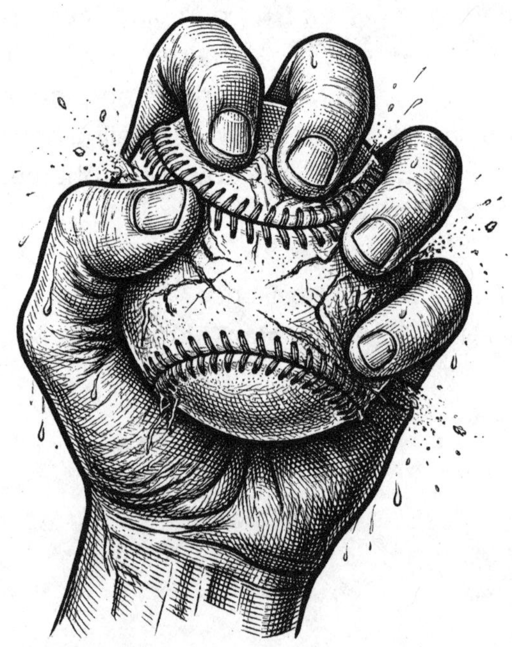

CHAPTER 3

ANXIETY

WHEN WORRY GRABS YOU BY THE BALLS

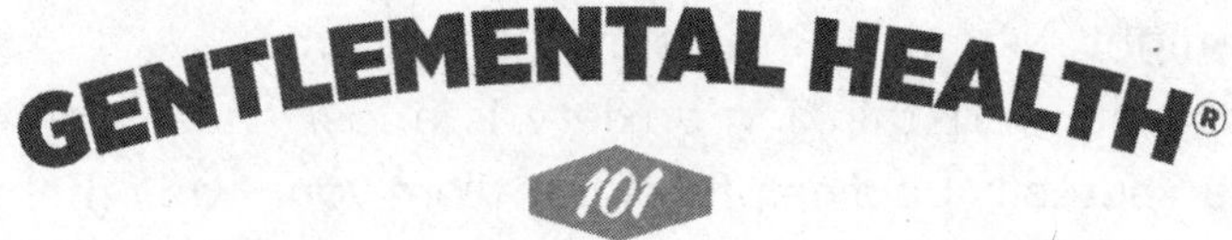

PICTURE THIS: it's 3 a.m. You're awake in bed for what feels like the fifteenth day in a row, staring wide-eyed at the ceiling. The only sound is the echo of your quickening pulse as your mind fast-tracks through life's worst-case scenarios. Even though there's no reason to believe that you face an imminent threat, you can't help fixating on the idea that there might just be something to those thoughts. Are your palms sweaty just thinking about it?

If this sounds familiar, you might be one of the millions of men impacted by anxiety. While it can be instinctual to laugh it off or believe it to be no big deal, unaddressed anxiety can trigger other negative outcomes, including chronic health issues, relationship breakdowns, impulsive behavior, substance misuse, and suicidal thoughts.

For starters, let's discuss the difference between stress and anxiety. Stress is typically triggered by external challenges or demands, like work deadlines, interpersonal conflicts, or financial stress. Given that stress is triggered by something external, it typically eases when that situation is resolved. This explains that whole-body feeling of relief when your loud-mouthed cubicle mate, Larry, finally decides to shove off for the day.

Anxiety, on the other hand, is an intense, persistent feeling of dread or unease about a threat that may or may not be present. While anxiety shows up similarly to stress in the body, it is a more persistent feeling that exists in a more-generalized fashion. This is why anxiety can cause us to start seeing life-or-death situations when there aren't any. And while your rational brain knows better, your sympathetic nervous system—which controls the fight-or-flight response—insists that it's go time.

Before you start thinking anxiety is a lost cause, remember that it can actually be a helpful signal from your body that something needs attention. Anxiety is an adaptive emotion and, believe it or not, you can use it to your advantage. Acknowledging anxiety affords you the opportunity to name it, take control of it, and build strategies to tackle it. There is a plethora of manly tools available, like confidence ladders (building small steps to face anxieties), Navy SEAL tactical breathing exercises, muscle relaxation techniques, shifting your cognitive perspective, or the ol' faithful—acknowledging and accepting that having anxiety f***ing sucks. If all else fails, you can try talking to a professional to start working towards an anxiety-free future.

Speaking of professionals, let's hear from Edmund Bourne to learn a little more about the X's and O's of anxiety and the best game plan to attack it.

LOOKING ANXIETY IN THE EYE

EDMUND BOURNE, PHD

You can better understand the nature of anxiety by looking at both what it is and what it is not. For example, anxiety can be distinguished from fear in several ways. When you are afraid, your fear is usually directed toward some concrete, external object or situation that is immediately present. You might fear not meeting a deadline, failing an exam, or being rejected by someone you want to please. When you experience anxiety, on the other hand, you frequently can't specify what it is you're anxious about.

Rather than fearing a specific object or situation, you may imagine some danger that is not immediately present and only remotely likely. You may be anxious about the future, about your overall safety or security, or about going forward in the face of uncertainty. Or you might be anxious about losing control of yourself or some situation. Or you might feel a vague anxiety about something bad happening when you face a specific challenge.

Anxiety affects your whole being. It is a physiological, behavioral, and psychological reaction all at once. On a physiological level, anxiety may include bodily reactions such as rapid heartbeat, muscle tension, queasiness, dry mouth, or sweating. On a behavioral level, it can paralyze your ability to act, express yourself, or deal with certain everyday situations. Psychologically, anxiety is a subjective state of apprehension and uneasiness. In its most extreme form, it can cause you to feel detached from yourself and even fearful of dying or going crazy.

The fact that anxiety can affect you on physiological, behavioral, and psychological levels has important implications for your attempts to cope. A complete program of coping with anxiety must address all three components. You need to learn how to reduce physiological reactivity, eliminate avoidance behavior, and change self-talk that perpetuates a state of apprehension and worry. Anxiety can appear in different forms and at different levels of intensity. It can range in severity from a mere twinge of uneasiness to a full-blown panic attack marked by heart palpitations, trembling, sweating, dizziness, disorientation, and terror. Anxiety that is not connected with any particular situation, that comes out of the blue, is called "free-floating anxiety" or, in more severe instances, a spontaneous "panic attack."

If your anxiety arises only in response to a specific situation, it is called "situational anxiety" or "phobic anxiety." Situational anxiety is different from everyday worries in that it tends to be out of proportion or unrealistic. If you have a disproportionate apprehension about driving on freeways, going to the doctor, or socializing, this may qualify as situational anxiety. Situational anxiety becomes phobic when you actually start to avoid the situation: if you give up driving on freeways, going to doctors, or socializing altogether. In other words, phobic anxiety is situational anxiety that includes persistent avoidance of the situation.

Often anxiety can be brought on merely by thinking about a particular situation. When you feel distressed about what might happen when you have to face a difficult or even phobic situation, you are experiencing what is called anticipatory anxiety. In its milder forms, anticipatory anxiety is indistinguishable from ordinary worry. Worrying can be defined as anticipating unpleas-ant consequences about a future situation. But sometimes antic-ipatory anxiety becomes intense enough to be anticipatory panic.

There is an important difference between spontaneous anxi-ety (or panic) and anticipatory anxiety (or panic). Spontaneous anxiety tends to come out of the blue, peaks to a high level very rapidly, and then subsides gradually. The peak is usually reached within five minutes, followed by a gradual tapering-off period of up to an hour or more. Anticipatory anxiety, on the other hand, tends to build up more gradually in response to encountering or simply thinking about a threatening situation, and may last longer. You may worry yourself into a frenzy about something for an hour or more and then let go of the worry as you tire or find something else to occupy your mind.

Causes of Anxiety

Anxiety symptoms often seem irrational and inexplicable, so it's only natural to raise the question, why?

Before considering in detail the various causes of anxiety, there are two general points you should bear in mind. First, although learning about the causes of anxiety can give you insight into how anxiety problems develop, such knowledge is unnecessary to overcome your particular difficulty. The various strategies for handling anxiety presented in this book, such as relaxation, realistic thinking, desensitization, exercise, nutrition, and self-nurturing, do not depend on a knowledge of underlying causes to be effective. However much you may know about causes, this knowledge is not necessarily what cures.

Second, be wary of the notion that there is one primary cause, or type of cause, for either everyday anxiety or anxiety disor-ders. Whether you are dealing with ordinary anxiety, apprehen-sion about a job interview, panic disorder, or obsessive-compulsive disorder, recognize that there is no one cause which, if removed, would eliminate the problem. Anxiety problems are brought about by a variety of causes operating on numerous levels. These levels include heredity, biology, family background and upbringing, conditioning, recent life changes, your self-talk and personal belief system, your ability to express feelings, current environmental stressors, and so on.

In sum, the idea that your particular difficulties are just a brain imbalance or just a psychological disturbance neglects the fact that nature and nurture are interactive. While brain imbalances may certainly be set up by heredity, they may also result from stress or psychological factors. Psychological problems, in turn, may be influenced by inborn biological predispositions. There is simply no way to say which came first or which is the "ultimate" cause. By the same token, a comprehensive approach to overcoming anxiety, panic, worry, or phobias cannot restrict itself to treating physiological or psychological causes in isolation. A variety of strategies dealing with several different levels—including biological, behavioral, emotional, mental, interpersonal, and even spiritual factors—are necessary. The causes of anxiety difficulties vary not only according to the level at which they occur, but also according to the time period over which they operate.

Finding the Anxiety "Off" Switch

From the time we awaken until we fall asleep, we are engaged in an almost constant mental bustle. Anxiety may accelerate this so that you feel like your mind is racing and you're bombarded with thoughts. This chapter introduces guided visualization, meditation, and other techniques that you can use daily to calm your mind and center yourself in the here and now. If you're like many Westerners, the idea of maintaining a daily regimen designed to relax your mind and induce serenity may sound foreign to you. But some of these techniques have endured for centuries and are now practiced the world over. In brief, they work.

Resisting or fighting anxiety is likely to make it worse. It's important to avoid tensing up in reaction to anxiety or trying to make it go away. Attempting to suppress or run away from the initial symptoms of anxiety is a way of telling yourself, "I can't handle it." A more constructive approach is to cultivate an attitude that says, "Okay, here it is again. I can allow my body to go through its reactions and handle this. I've done it before." Acceptance of anxiety symptoms is the key. By cultivating an attitude of acceptance in the face of anxiety, you allow it to move through and pass. Anxiety is caused by a sudden surge of adrenaline. If you can let go and allow your body to have its reactions (such as heart palpitations, chest constriction, sweaty palms, and dizziness) caused by this surge, it will pass soon. Most of the adrenaline released will be metabolized and reabsorbed within five minutes. As soon as this happens, you'll start to feel better. Anxiety reactions are time limited. In most cases, anxiety peaks and begins to subside within a few minutes. Some anxiety may persist for a while, but the worst is over in a short time. It will pass more quickly if you don't aggravate it by fighting against it or reacting to it with fearful self-talk beginning with "What if…"

Acceptance of the initial symptoms of anxiety is very important, but then it's time to do something. Anxiety and worry are passive states where you feel vulnerable, out of control, or even paralyzed. If you stand still and do nothing, your anxiety may tend to maintain itself or even build, leaving you feeling victimized. When anxiety comes on, always accept it first, then realize that there are many things you can actively do to redirect the energy spent on the anxiety into something constructive. In short, don't try to fight with anxiety, but don't do nothing either.

To cope with anxiety in the moment, there are three types of recommended activities:

- Coping strategies, which are active techniques to offset anxiety or distract yourself from it.

- Coping statements, which are mental techniques designed to redirect your mind away from and replace fearful self-talk.

- Affirmations, which can be used much like coping statements but are intended to work over a longer time period. Coping strategies and statements help to get you through a particular episode of anxiety, while affirmations work with changing your core beliefs. For example, you could use a particular coping strategy or statement to get through a difficult situation, and you could also bring to mind an affirmation about freedom from fear you have been working with for months.

EXPERIENCE SOMETHING IMMEDIATELY PLEASURABLE

Just as anger and anxiety are incompatible responses, so the feeling of pleasure is incompatible with an anxiety state.

Any of the following may help to offset anxiety, worry, or even panic:

- Have your significant other or spouse hold you (or give you a back rub)

- Take a hot shower or relax in a hot bath

- Have a pleasurable snack or meal

- Engage in sexual activity

- Read humorous books or watch a comical video

TRY A COGNITIVE SHIFT

Thinking about any of the following ideas may help you to shift your point of view so that you can let go of worry or anxious thoughts:

- Acknowledge that it would be okay to lighten up about this.

- Turn the problem over to your Higher Power.

- Trust in the inevitability of it passing. Affirm "this too will pass."

- Realize that it's not likely to be as bad as your worst thoughts about it.

- Realize that working with the problem is part of your path to healing and recovery.

- Remember not to blame yourself. You're doing your best, and that's the best anyone can do.

- Expand your compassion for all people who experience similar anxiety. Remember you're not alone.

GENERAL COPING STATEMENTS FOR ANXIETY OR PANIC

- I can handle these symptoms or sensations.

- These sensations (feelings) are just a reminder to use my coping skills.

- I can take my time and allow these feelings to pass. I deserve to feel okay right now.

- This is just adrenaline—it will pass in a few minutes. This will pass soon.

- I can ride this through.

- These are just thoughts—not reality.

- This is just anxiety—I'm not going to let it get to me. This anxiety won't hurt me, even if it doesn't feel good. Nothing about these sensations or feelings is dangerous.

- I don't need to let these feelings and sensations stop me. I can continue to function.

- This isn't dangerous.

- These are just (anxious) thoughts—nothing more. So what.

PUT YOUR COPING STATEMENTS ON CARDS

So that your coping statements are readily available, it's a good idea to put your favorite ones on an index card (or several cards, if you prefer), which you can keep in your wallet or tape to the dashboard of your car. Whenever you feel symptoms of anxiety coming on, bring out the card and read it. Remember, you need to practice your coping statements many times before you'll fully internalize them. Eventually, they will take the place of the fearful, catastrophic self-talk that tends to keep your anxiety going. The effort you put into practicing coping statements will be well worth it.

AFFIRMATIONS

Coping statements, along with the coping strategies discussed earlier, can help diminish anxiety in the moment. Affirmations can be in the moment, but are also useful over the long term. They can help you to change long-standing beliefs which tend to perpetuate anxiety. Their purpose is to help you cultivate a more constructive and self-empowering attitude toward your own experience of anxiety. Instead of being a passive victim of anxiety, you can cultivate an attitude of active mastery. Instead of feeling helplessly stuck or overwhelmed by panic, fearfulness, or worry, you can cultivate an attitude of greater confidence and faith in your ability to overcome your anxiety.

NEGATIVE THOUGHTS AND POSITIVE AFFIRMATIONS TO COMBAT THEM

- This is unbearable.
+ I can learn how to cope better with this.

- What if this goes on without letting up?
+ I'll deal with this one day at a time. I don't have to project into the future.

- I feel damaged, inadequate relative to others.
+ Some of us have steeper paths to walk than others. That doesn't make me less valuable as a human being—even if I accomplish less in the outer world.

- Why do I have to deal with this? Other people seem freer to enjoy their lives.
+ Life is a school. For whatever reasons, at least for now, I've been given a steeper path—a tougher curriculum. That doesn't make

me wrong. In fact, adversity develops qualities of strength and compassion.

- Having this condition seems unfair.
+ Life can appear unfair from a human perspective. If we could see the bigger picture, we'd see that everything is proceeding according to plan.

- I don't know how to cope with this.
+ I can learn to cope better, step by step—with this and any difficulty life brings.

- I feel so inadequate relative to others.
+ Let people do what they do in the outer world. I'm following a path of inner growth and transformation, which is at least equally valuable. Finding peace in myself can be a gift to others.

- Each day seems like a major challenge.
+ I'm learning to take things more slowly. I make time to take care of myself. I make time to do small things to nurture myself.

- I don't understand why I'm this way—why this happened to me.
+ The causes are many, including heredity, early environment, and cumulative stress. Understanding causes satisfies the intellect, but it's not what heals.

- I feel like I'm going crazy.
+ When anxiety is high, I feel like I'm losing control. But that feeling has nothing to do with going crazy. Anxiety disorders are a long way from the category of disorders labeled "crazy."

- I have to really fight this.
+ Struggling with a problem won't help as much as making more time in my life to better care for myself.

- I shouldn't have let this happen to me.
+ The long-term causes of this problem lie in heredity and childhood environment, so I didn't cause this condition. I can now take responsibility for getting better.

Things Your Body Can Do to Shrug It Off

Anxiety often manifests itself as a cluster of physical symptoms. In fact, when asked to describe their anxiety, many people begin by enumerating a list of disquieting physical sensations, such as shortness of breath, muscle tension, hyperventilation, and palpitations. Such symptoms reinforce anxiety-producing thoughts. Try to think for a moment of your anxiety as a solely physical condition. What are the symptoms of this condition? How do they affect your sense of well-being? How do you respond to them? Although it may seem like these physical symptoms are automatic reflexes beyond your control, you can take comfort in knowing that they are not. With practice, you can stem the physical effects of anxiety and free yourself from its grip.

PROGRESSIVE MUSCLE RELAXATION

Progressive muscle relaxation is a simple technique used to halt anxiety by relaxing your muscles one group at a time. Its effectiveness was recognized decades ago by Edmund Jacobson, a Chicago physician. In 1929 he published what has become a classic, *Progressive Relaxation*. In it he described this deep muscle relaxation technique which, he asserted, required no imagination, willpower, or suggestion. His technique is based on the premise that the body responds to anxiety-inducing thoughts with muscle tension. This muscle tension then induces more anxiety and triggers a vicious cycle. Stop the muscle tension, stop the cycle. "An anxious mind cannot exist in a relaxed body," Dr. Jacobson once said.

"I'M UPTIGHT"

If your anxiety is strongly associated with muscle tension, progressive muscle relaxation will probably prove an especially useful tool for you. This muscle tension is often what leads you to say that you are "uptight" or "tense." You may experience chronic tightness in your shoulders and neck, for example, which can be effectively relieved by practicing progressive muscle relaxation. Other symptoms that respond well to progressive muscle relaxation include tension headaches, backaches, tightness in the jaw, tightness around the eyes, muscle spasms, high blood pressure, and insomnia. If you are troubled by racing thoughts, you may find that systematically relaxing your muscles tends to slow down your mind. If you take tranquilizers, you may find that regular practice of progressive muscle relaxation will enable you to lower your dosage.

CUE-CONTROLLED RELAXATION

In cue-controlled relaxation, you learn to relax your muscles whenever you want by combining a verbal suggestion with abdominal breathing. First, take a comfortable position, then release as much tension as you can using the relaxation-without-tension method. Focus on your belly as it moves in and out with each breath. Make breaths slow and rhythmic. With each breath let yourself become more and more relaxed. Now, on every inhalation say to yourself the words *breathe in*, and as you exhale, the word *relax*. Just keep saying to yourself, "Breathe in ... relax, breathe in ... relax," while letting go of tension throughout your body. Continue this practice for five minutes, repeating the key phrases with each breath.

The cue-controlled method teaches your body to associate the word "relax" with the feeling of relaxation. After you have practiced this technique for a while and the association is strong, you'll be able to relax your muscles anytime, anywhere, just by mentally repeating, "Breathe in ... relax," and by releasing any feelings of tightness throughout your body. Cue-controlled relaxation can give you stress relief in less than a minute.

ABDOMINAL BREATHING

Most of us don't think much about our breathing patterns and how they reflect and contribute to our emotional state. But the way you breathe directly reflects the level of tension you carry in your body and can aggravate or diminish your anxiety symptoms. If you are like many anxiety sufferers, you've experienced one or both of the following breathing problems:

- Breathing too high up in your chest, with your breathing too shallow.

- Breathing rapidly or hyperventilation, which results in breathing out too much carbon dioxide relative to the amount of oxygen carried in your bloodstream.

Is your breath slow or rapid? Deep or shallow? Does it center around a point high in your chest or down in your abdomen? You might also take note of changes in your breathing pattern under stress compared to when you are more relaxed.

CHEST BREATHING VERSUS ABDOMINAL BREATHING

Under tension, your breathing usually becomes shallow and rapid, and occurs high in the chest. Shallow, chest-level breathing, when rapid, can lead to hyperventilation. Hyperventilation, in turn, can cause physical symptoms associated with anxiety, such as light-headedness, dizziness, heart palpitations, or tingling sensations. When relaxed, you breathe more fully, more deeply, and from your abdomen. It's difficult to be tense and to breathe from your abdomen at the same time. By changing your breathing pattern from up in your chest to down in your abdomen (stomach area), you can reverse the cycle and transform your breathing into a built-in tool for anxiety control.

Abdominal breathing triggers a host of physiological transactions that promote relaxation and diminish anxiety. Listed below are some of the benefits of abdominal breathing that translate into greater relaxation and lowered anxiety.

- Increased oxygen supply to the brain and musculature.

- Stimulation of the parasympathetic nervous system. This branch of your autonomic nervous system promotes a state of calmness and quiescence. It works in a fashion exactly opposite to the sympathetic branch of your nervous system, which stimulates a state of emotional arousal and the very physiological reactions underlying panic or anxiety.

- Greater feelings of connectedness between your mind and body. Anxiety and worry tend to keep you up in your head. A few minutes of deep abdominal breathing will help bring you down into your whole body.

- More efficient excretion of bodily toxins. Many toxic substances in the body are excreted through the lungs.

- Improved concentration. If your mind is racing, it's difficult to focus your attention. Abdominal breathing helps to quiet your mind.

- Abdominal breathing by itself can trigger a relaxation response.

The exercises below will help you change your breathing pattern. By practicing them, you can achieve a state of deep relaxation in a short period of time. Just three minutes of practicing abdominal breathing or the calming breath exercise will usually induce a deep state of relaxation. Many people successfully use one or the other technique to abort a panic attack at its first stirrings. The techniques are also very helpful in diminishing anticipatory anxiety you may experience in advance of facing a fearful situation or in easing everyday worry.

STEPS FOR ABDOMINAL BREATHING

1. Note the level of tension you're feeling. Then place one hand on your abdomen, right beneath your rib cage.

2. Inhale slowly and deeply through your nose into the bottom of your lungs; in other words, send the air as low down as you can. If you're breathing from your abdomen, your hand should actually rise. Your chest should move only slightly while your abdomen expands.

3. When you've taken in a full breath, pause for a moment and then exhale slowly through your nose or mouth, depending on your preference. Be sure to exhale fully. As you exhale, allow your whole body to just let go (you might visualize your arms and legs going loose and limp like a rag doll).

4. Do ten slow, full abdominal breaths. Try to keep your breathing smooth and regular, without gulping in a big breath or letting your breath out all at once. It will help to slow down

your breathing if you slowly count to four on the inhale and then slowly count to four on the exhale. Use this count to slow down your breathing for a few breaths, then let it go. Remember to pause briefly at the end of each inhalation.

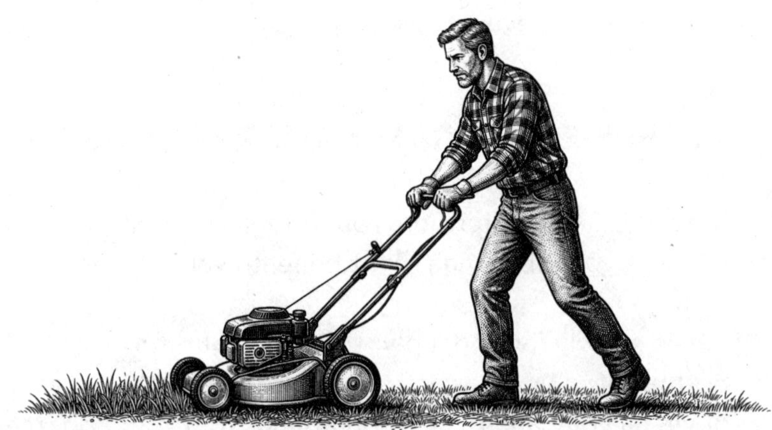

Dr. Rich's Anxiety Remedy: Mow the Lawn

Nothing soothes a man's spirit quite like the hut-one-hut-two pacing of guiding a mower in picture-perfect diamond patterns across the yard. It turns out that mowing perennial ryegrass is like combining meditation with gas-powered engines. It's mind-blowing.

Want more manly tips on Anxiety? Explore the Gentlemental Health card on **ManTherapy.org**.

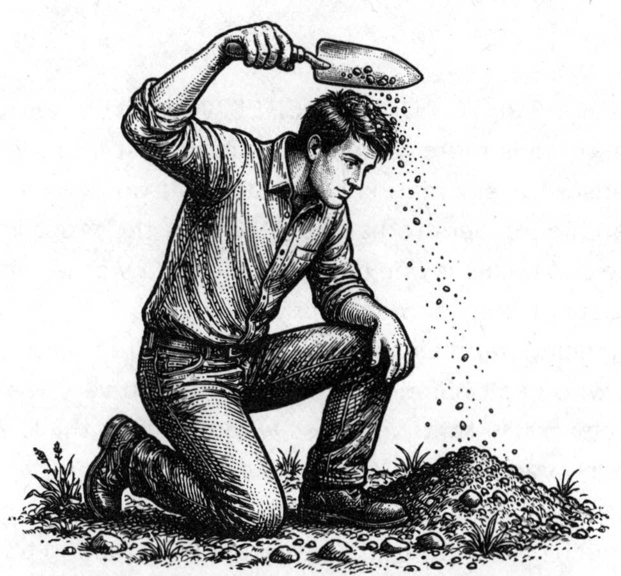

CHAPTER 4

DEPRESSION

YOU CAN'T RUB DIRT ON YOUR FEELINGS

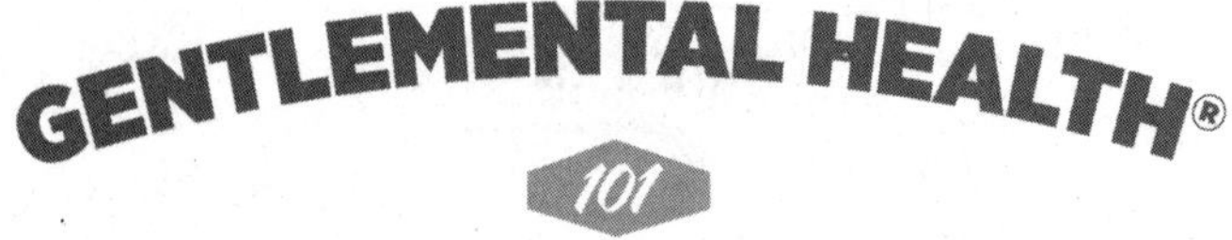

WE'RE NOT HERE TO PULL PUNCHES. When it comes to mental health, nothing is more important than honest, frank conversation to ensure every man knows what he's up against and has clear marching orders to handle it. One of the most important topics we can tackle is one that underlies many other challenges and impacts millions of men—depression.

Experiencing depression doesn't mean you're a namby-pamby crybaby who can't handle life. Depression is a very real change in brain chemistry that can mess with how you think, feel, and show up in everyday life. It looks like having an empty tank for the things you care about, losing interest in your passions, sleeping too much or too little, changes in appetite (eating too little or eating your feelings), struggles with focus, isolating from loved ones, or even thinking that life isn't worth living.

For many men, depression doesn't necessarily present as "sad," but often shows up as irritability, anger, or numbness. It can lead to physical problems like headaches, gut issues, and increased discomfort, as well as a decline in work performance and abandoning life goals. To put it bluntly: if unaddressed, depression can wreak havoc on one's quality of life.

However, there's a difference between proactively dealing with depression and masking feelings. Camouflage might come in handy when stalking a 12-point buck through the woods. But camouflage behaviors like overworking, excessive drinking or drug use, gambling, porn addiction, or impulsive behavior only serve to punt a man's problems downfield and don't address the beast hiding in plain sight.

The good news is that depression doesn't have to be the boogeyman lurking in the corner. There are a range of tactics you can use to positively impact your well-being, which we'll explore in the coming pages. However, if intense feelings persist, reach out to a professional for help diagnosing what's going on and zeroing in on other treatment options.

Remember: there are many shades of blue when it comes to depression, and you don't need to have full-blown "major depressive disorder" to experience symptoms and benefit from these interventions. As any craftsman knows, it's all about finding the right tools you need to get the job done.

If you're ready to hop to it and start rising above what's getting you down, let's explore some manly strategies for dealing with depression from another expert, Randy Patterson.

WHEN MISERY SNEAKS UP ON YOU

RANDY J. PATTERSON, PHD

Many years ago, I was midway through my predoctoral internship in psychology when misery popped by for what turned out to be a yearlong visit.

At first I had no idea what was happening. I couldn't sleep, I couldn't eat, I could barely read a sentence, and a flight of stairs might just as well have been the Annapurna Circuit. Nothing appealed. At times, it seemed I could barely talk. Once, in a depressive fog, I greeted a new patient with the pronouncement, "This is Randy Paterson," causing the poor woman to peer around to see if I might be introducing her to someone more promising than I was.

A flippant list of a few symptoms does not serve to illuminate the sheer wretchedness of much of this period. I could go on, but let's leave that for another day.

I was treating depression, for goodness' sake, and still failed to notice it overtaking me. When I finally twigged, I was tempted to dismiss it. Young, healthy, pursuing a career I'd chosen at the age of eight—what did I have to be so unhappy about?

The answers, rolling their eyes, eventually tapped me on the shoulder, annoyed that I hadn't noticed them standing there.

Some were outside my control. The internship demanded long hours on multiple wards, seeing patients with both psychiatric and physical illnesses, many of the latter being terminal cases. One of my best friends at the time was dying. My internship was far from the friends I'd developed in graduate school, in a bedroom community known chiefly for the cheerful ease with which the residents had evacuated some years before when a train carrying toxic chemicals derailed. (The miracle, so the local joke went, was not that everyone got out but that they ever returned.)

Some of the factors, however, were the result of my own choices. I didn't need to work quite as much as I did, and I was pushing myself in the evenings and on weekends to write my dissertation. I was drinking far too much coffee and eating too much gelatinous hospital food. I wasn't staying in contact with friends, seldom left my slum apartment (in a neighborhood that was red-circled by the social workers at the hospital), and got almost no exercise.

I scraped through, largely by fantasizing that I was my own patient and (mostly) following the standard recommendations. I exercised more, cut the coffee, took weekends off, ate better, made a point of seeing friends, and so on. Still, it took almost a year before I was back to what I usually considered my normal state.

After graduation, I specialized in the treatment of anxiety disorders, coyly shying away from seeing too much in the way of depression. A bit too close to home for comfort. Homesick for mountains, I applied for every possible job on the West Coast and (fate having a delicious sense of humor) was offered a position as coordinator of a hospital-based mood disorder program. I accepted and, contrary to my own predictions, stayed there for nine years before opening a private clinic with a focus on—you can guess—mood problems. Our hospital team ran groups for people in the grip of more than just garden-variety misery. All had been hospitalized; most of them, several times. Their struggle easily dwarfed anything I had gone though. In my own cushioned life, I had visited the edge of the valley, but clearly had not dropped to its very bottom.

Early on, we began conducting a discussion exercise as part of the first session of the program. Our clients had been struggling to feel better for months—in some cases, for decades. They were understandably skeptical that anything we might do in our little group would be helpful. So we turned it around.

"Imagine that you could earn $10 million for just half an hour's work—let's say tomorrow morning between 11:00 and 11:30. All you would have to do is make yourself feel worse than you do now. Worse, in fact, than you've felt in the past week. How would you do it?"

Sometimes people would object, saying that it still wouldn't be worth the money or that they feared getting stuck there. One woman gazed balefully across the table at me. "So far, I have been doing this for free. Ten million? Fine."

What ensued, invariably, was a free-for-all of ideas that came haltingly at first and then in a flood. After one session, a hospital cleaner stopped in the hall as I was locking up and asked what had been going on in there. "Depression group," I said. "But they were laughing," she said, frowning. "You don't hear a lot of laughter in this building."

Each time we did the exercise, however, the humor would subside when I asked, "When you wake up in the morning, and you're already miserable, what do you feel like doing?" They would begin listing many of the same things that they had just nominated as strategies to feel worse.

"Why do you think that is?"

Some worried that perhaps they just liked being depressed. But this didn't fit. Of all the experiences they'd had, depression was almost always the most wretched. They didn't like it at all.

Misery changes everything. It affects how we feel, how we think, what we do—and it alters our impulses. When we are miserable, we are usually tempted to do precisely what, at other times, we know will make it worse. The result can be that we appear to be bringing on our own discomfort.

"In this group," I and the other leaders would say, "we're going to try to become aware of these impulses—and often we're going to try to do the opposite. Most of what we talk about won't seem tempting or promising or even logical. The strategies may feel wrong. But what feels right when you're miserable is what feeds the misery, not what feeds you."

The Difference Between Feeling "Off" and Depression

Clinical depression, as should be obvious, is an extreme form of human misery. But there is no clear border dividing it from its milder cousins. Many of my present-day clients are less than happy about their lives, but not clinically depressed. Some arrive at my office doing just fine—but having heard about the new field of positive psychology, they wonder if they can go from tolerable or middling life satisfaction to better than average. Some of the strategies are unique to where a person starts out. Most are not.

We can learn from the answers given by the truly depressed to the Ten-Million-Dollar Question. Indeed, most of the strategies in this chapter first arose in those groups. You can ask the question of yourself. If you wanted to feel worse rather than better, what would you do?

Misery is a normal human experience. We all encounter it to varying degrees, and often we are surprised by its knock. So rather than waiting, let's open the door and set out to find it. A misery safari. Pith helmets are optional.

How Do You Know If You Have It?

What causes a person's mood to rise or fall? Apart from mysterious fluctuations in the internal soup in which our brains simmer, what factors launch a person upward to the pinnacles of happiness or propel them to the valley floor?

We can divide the answers into two categories.

The first—let's call it Column A—comprises the inventory of catastrophe that can overtake us. Despite our privileged society, tragedy and disappointment still exist. Cars collide. Cells metastasize. Industries fail. Bodies age. Partners leave. Friends move. Roofs leak. Poverty and disease still thrive. We are not in full control of the circumstances of our lives. We can imagine that we have arranged our lives so carefully, with such foresight, that we have assured our happiness—and yet we know that circumstance can sweep it all away.

So there are limits to our personal influence. We can do all the right things and still get hit by a bus. If we are five feet tall, we can practice and perfect our basketball skills all we like, but we will still never play in the NBA. We can eat right, give up smoking, and take our vitamins, and we are still guaranteed to slip off the dish before our 120th birthday.

Life can impose a dizzying array of circumstances upon us that may limit our happiness or create misery: war, poverty, refugee status, personal misfortune of any stripe. You may be born with any of a variety of constraints—sensory, intellectual, social, familial. We can be fired, dumped, duped, flooded, infected, bombed, bullied, struck, abandoned, bankrupted, blind-sided, T-boned, or poisoned by an undercooked hamburger.

Some events, in retrospect, seem to have been so unlikely that it never occurred to you to worry about them. Just when my own life was going pretty well, I was shot off my bicycle by a deer that had been struck and air-launched by a passing vehicle. Sometimes it appears that fate has it in for you. I took my deer impact as a message from the fates to make some much-needed changes in my career. "Look what we can do! Get on with your life, or next time it'll be a moose."

In addition to these capricious whims of fate, however, there are many influences on our moods that lie within our own control. Let's put these in Column B. We can choose what to eat, how to spend our time, how much exercise to get, and what to make priorities in our lives. All of these will influence—within the limits fate imposes upon us—how happy or miserable we become. We may not be able to live to be a thousand years old no matter what we do, but we can increase the likelihood of reaching a relatively healthy ninety. Whatever our lifespan, we can choose to spend our years isolated in front of a computer monitor or fully engaged with humanity and existence.

Even the factors outside our control may not impose limits that are as rigid as they appear. Some who have gone through horrific tribulations or who labor under what we might imagine to be intolerable circumstances are, despite it all, fairly happy. We might imagine that we could never again be upbeat if our partner left us or if we lost our job or if our home burned down. But read any number of biographies, and you find people who have gone through unimaginable losses and eventually returned to a full emotional life. We too may be surprised by joy just when all chance of it seems to have been extinguished.

There's no point in sitting in a field either summoning or attempting to avert an asteroid strike. The events of Column A are out of our control. We will take as given the fact that every one of us has circumstances that are immutable and unwelcome. Our efforts will instead focus on Column B: the mood-influencing factors that lie within the scope of our own choices. Within this chapter, we will examine elements of life that can be controlled or selected, for good or ill. There are many in the world who might look at the comfort, luxury, and leisure of life in developed countries and assume that misery would be impossible in such a place. Surely there is a lower limit to how awful a person can feel when the refrigerator is full. This appears not to be the case, however. As the data on life satisfaction, depression, and suicide all attest, no amount of wealth or good fortune can entirely prevent misery. Our species has a talent for it.

If you are struggling through a wilderness and run up against an impenetrable wall, it only makes sense to look around and try the other direction. Given the thousands of books pointing toward happiness and their apparent lack of impact on global life satisfaction, perhaps we should turn our attention to the almost empty shelf nearby, the one reserved for guideposts to another destination: misery. If, in the presence of unparalleled wealth and privilege, we are capable of dissatisfaction, then perhaps misery is humanity's true signature strength. Let's optimize it.

This chapter then, strikes off in the opposite direction to all those guides to the alleged good life. If we embrace misery as our goal, what is the path? Given the rarity of guides to this twilit land, one might think there would be little research to guide us. In fact, nothing could be further from the truth. Millions—perhaps billions—of dollars have been spent researching the question of how people become miserable. Today, if we want to be unhappy, we know how to bring it about. We have the technology.

Perhaps you are undecided about this quest. No matter. People buy travel guides all the time and never visit the regions covered. You need not sign a declaration in blood that you will commit to the path. But, in case one day you should choose this adventure, let's describe the route.

Ways to Feel Worse and Never Get Back on Track

One of the great paradoxes about lowering your mood is that it often works best to strike out in the direction of happiness rather than aiming straight at misery. The quest for uplift often hides a stairway leading sharply downward.

The use of a chemical assist to raise one's mood is a classic example. People drink alcohol, smoke pot, and practice other forms of "informal pharmacy" largely to elevate the mood. In the short term, these substances often perform precisely as advertised. In the long run, however, the diligent user can reap a substantial harvest in unhappiness.

Despite our culture's tendency to cluck disapprovingly about self-medication to alter mood, the most widely used drug is both legal and socially acceptable: alcohol. It causes more deaths (both directly, via organ damage, and indirectly, through traffic fatalities and other mishaps) than any other drug of abuse. Population-wide, it also creates the most misery. Moderate consumption of one to two drinks per day, however, appears to be relatively benign for most people. This is unlikely to assist you to your goal unless you have a familial vulnerability to alcohol dependence, in which case any use at all can help you find the fabled slippery slope.

For the maximum effect, you will want to drink more than a glass of wine with dinner. Alcohol is a depressant, so even if it affects no other aspect of your life, it will insidiously begin downshifting your mood.

The overuse of alcohol can have an impact on all areas of your life. For example, it tends to anesthetize the inhibitory pathways of the brain. This is one of its biggest attractions for the shy. They can relax, open up, converse more easily, and drop rigid boundaries (and sometimes clothes). The hidden benefit for our purposes is that inhibition is critically important for proper functioning in social settings. We may feel tempted to make fun of a friend's outfit or political opinions, but normally we refrain from doing so. With overuse—and it's always difficult to calculate the ideal dose just so—alcohol will take the brakes off the mouth, allowing us to career downhill into the realm of the social pariah.

Further, alcohol reduces the capacity for self-reflection. Under its influence, we may think we are performing well at work, being funny at a party, and driving with perfect skill—but we're not.

One of the reasons that people are not more miserable than they are is that, sober, they instinctively respond to feedback and hold themselves back when they see they are coloring outside the lines. Given enough alcohol, however, we can no longer detect the lines and so push fearlessly beyond them.

Longer term, the pinball of alcohol dependence can carom off of any of life's surfaces, intensifying and accelerating at every step. It can impair career success, friendships, marriages, child raising, the deeper stages of sleep, finances, and almost any other aspect of an otherwise-fulfilling life.

What about other drugs? This book is far too brief to describe the myriad downward possibilities offered by each substance on the prohibition list. Broadly speaking, however, the pattern is similar to that for alcohol—with the added bonus of illegality and all of the fun and consequences that can bring.

There is one more substance worth considering, however, and it is again a legal one: caffeine. Sharp observers in North America have noted the increase in urban coffee shop density over the past few decades, concluding that if the pace continues there will be no room for any other form of business within twenty years.

Caffeine can trigger a stress response with the attendant fight-or-flight flavors of unhappiness: anger and anxiety. Small doses, for most people, do not seem significant and may only serve to sharpen concentration and motivation. But once one graduates to a more heroic habit (as little as three cups of drip coffee per day), anxiety, anger, or both are likely to be accentuated. You may even be able to trigger panic attacks or outbursts of rage. More often, you will experience a grinding uneasiness and irritability.

Plus, if you drink enough—of either coffee or alcohol—you will always have to be within 150 yards of a bathroom.

SET VAPID GOALS

One of the best ways to be miserable is to relinquish your goals altogether, thus becoming utterly directionless. But if, like many people, misery is not your only goal, then you can dissatisfy yourself with the way you approach your various missions.

Goal setting involves the creation of two categories of ambition. Ultimate goals are the end points of the process: learning Spanish, having a tidy garage, settling on a career, completing a school program, creating a social network, bench pressing two hundred pounds. Ask people about their own goals, and virtually everything they say will be an ultimate goal.

Immediate goals are the small steps in service to an ultimate goal. So if your ultimate goal is to complete your income tax form, then spending twenty minutes gathering the paperwork might be your first immediate goal. If the ultimate goal is to move to Scranton, an immediate goal might be to visit a real estate website for that city.

The cause of misery is well served by failure. So it's important to ignore the so-called SMART rules, which dictate that effective immediate goals should be:

- **Specific.** You know how you will accomplish the task. "Take the number 19 bus to the Aquatic Center."

- **Measurable.** You will know whether or not you have succeeded. "Get in pool and swim one lap."

- **Action-oriented.** Your goal is to do something, not to think or feel a particular way. "Swim the lap—even if I hate it and think my bathing cap looks stupid."

- **Realistic.** You already know you can do it, even if you don't feel particularly well. "I could swim twenty laps not long ago; I'm absolutely certain I can swim at least one."

- **Time-defined.** You have a clear time frame for completion of the goal within the coming week. "On Thursday evening."

These rules make success more likely, resulting in increased motivation and interest in the succeeding steps. This only means that you will be more likely to get up off that comfortable couch and continue working on your project. Instead, make all of your immediate goals VAPID:

- **Vague.** You should be unclear how you are going to complete the goal. If you want to cross-country ski, you should forget all about looking into lessons, thinking about how to get there, or ensuring you have the right clothing.

- **Amorphous.** The finish line for your immediate goal should be indistinct, so your depressive self can disqualify any progress you have made. Setting a goal to "work on the back garden," for example, allows you to criticize yourself for not finishing everything, thus eliminating any of the satisfaction you might otherwise feel.

- **Pie in the sky.** Indulge your innate ability to overestimate what you can do. Say that today you will paint the entire house or revamp your company's finances. With the ensuing failure, you will be able to beat yourself up about your incompetence.

- **Irrelevant.** Tell yourself that if you achieve your ultimate goal of overcoming social anxiety, you will once again be able to visit your bank. You should therefore lock yourself at home studying investment strategy as a "necessary" prerequisite.

- **Delayed.** Avoid setting a specific time for the completion of your goal. Instead, resolve to get to work the moment you "feel like it." Because it is vanishingly unlikely that you will ever feel like re-caulking the bathroom tile, you can ensure that it will never be done.

Regardless of whether you set SMART or VAPID immediate goals, you can ensure disappointment by—as usual—the simple expedient of following the injunctions of the culture. In this case, keeping your eye on the ball.

Set your ultimate goal (say, to find a long-term relationship), break it down into smaller steps (join the rowing club, accept the invitation to the departmental party, purchase non-droopy underwear), and then, no matter what happens with those immediate goals, continue to hold your attention relentlessly on the ultimate goal.

Most ultimate goals are a long way off—hence the need to break them down into smaller steps. You might achieve them only once, and only after a great deal of effort. If you allow yourself to focus on the immediate goals, you will frequently find that you have succeeded. *Hey, look—I actually smiled at the cute barista.* This runs the risk of increasing your enthusiasm for the path you have created for yourself.

Instead, by stubbornly attending to the ultimate goal (Have I got a partner yet?), the discouraging answer (Well, no) will recur again and again and again. If there are fifty steps in the process, you will get forty-nine identical answers of "not yet." You can maintain the aura of failure for almost the entire journey. And because this continual discouragement will degrade your interest and motivation, you are likely to give up long before you reach the success of your ultimate goal, thus making the sense of failure permanent.

DUTY FIRST, LIFE LATER

"I haven't seen a movie or read a novel since I got here."

A group of us were chatting in the hall of the psychology

department, preparing for our weekly departure to the student pub. Sharon (as I'll call her) had stopped by briefly. She wouldn't be going, of course. Too busy. She was always too busy. No one was skeptical of her claim. She had never been seen at a social event in the year since our cohort started the program. She said she'd be able to relax once her master's thesis was defended.

Once that goal was accomplished, leisure continued to recede. She would relax once she had finished collecting her PhD data, once her comprehensive examinations were over, once she defended her dissertation, once she'd completed her year of postdoctoral supervision.

I haven't seen her in many years, but she's always been there in the back of my mind. I've wondered if she's still at it. Once I've published some articles. Once I've gotten a promotion. Once my private practice is running. Once the mortgage is paid off. Once I retire. Then my life will start. Unless something else gets in the way.

The Marshmallow Test is an assessment of a child's ability to delay gratification. The experimenter presents the child with a marshmallow and announces that she will be back in fifteen minutes. If the marshmallow hasn't been eaten at that point, the child can have a second one.

Children vary in their ability to sit in front of the marshmallow and not eat it. Some give in immediately, while others squirm in agonies of temptation. It turns out that the simple binary outcome (eaten or not) is nicely predictive of later academic success. Delayers generally do better. It's easy to see why. Success depends to a great extent on a person's ability to study when they could be watching television and to work their way through the boring bits of otherwise interesting projects.

Adults sometimes respond to a description of the test with a sigh of ennui. "I don't like marshmallows anyway, so I don't see the relevance." Swap out the marshmallow with the grown-up equivalent, however, and watch the fun. Lift the cover and reveal a plate of chocolate. A line of cocaine. A bottle of scotch. A pornographic video. A television remote. A couch. Suddenly the test isn't quite so hypothetical. Leave them for fifteen minutes, and only the crumbs remain.

The ability to delay gratification is a double-edged sword, with misery lying seductively on both sides. Too little self-discipline, and we accomplish nothing, wallowing in our consumption. Too much, and we can choke the joy out of our lives. It is only along the narrow flat of the blade that happiness-inducing moderation can be found. This tightrope is easily avoided. If you become especially adept at passing the Marshmallow Test, you may suppress even your better aspirations in favor of conformity to the expectations or wishes of others. You may also become so focused on a single, genuinely held goal (like becoming a respected professional) that your life becomes imbalanced. You may spend no time socializing with friends, enjoying life, or doing any of the things that sustain you for the long haul. Even if you can keep the flame of your passion burning, you may find that you have realized one life goal (such as career success) but missed out on all the others.

You can choose to push most of your goals or pleasures into the future, telling yourself that there will always be time for them later. Relationships, novels, travel, experiences, contributions to the world. Dinner with friends. Playing with the cat. Walking in the forest. Even a night at the pub. It may turn out that the future is shorter than you thought it would be. And when "later" appears, if it ever does, you may have forgotten what your plans were, or what your life was meant to be about. You will no longer know how to have fun, how to lie in a hammock, how to be a friend, how to raise your children. You will only remember how to be working, working, working.

Sharon would have passed the Marshmallow Test with no difficulty. I think I would have too—as a child, I still had uneaten Halloween candy in January. But I had the example of a father who delayed gratification constantly, apparently believing that he would start living his life when he retired—something he died before doing. So in graduate school I went to the pub, I saw movies,

I read books, and I had relationships. I lived my life, knowing that the future was an imaginary construct that might not exist.

Don't use me as your model: I wasn't trying to be unhappy. That, when it happened, was accidental. Instead, use Sharon. If you have a sense of what you would like your life to be about, set that insight aside. Tell yourself that you have more important things to think about right now—like completing your degree or getting your career established or paying off the mortgage. Right now you have to work hard. You are sacrificing for a distant future. If the present does not seem very enjoyable, that's all right. The future will be all the rosier for it.

Tell yourself that when you just reach that next hurdle, you'll be able to sit back, relax, and work on your life's purpose. There's plenty of time. You can get to it when your to-do list runs out. Become a supreme delayer of gratification. Push your life endlessly into the future. Forget balance. Hang on to the marshmallow long enough, and it will become inedible.

It's important to suppress any awareness of the tendency to fix your eyes on a new hurdle when you pass the previous one. Just keep going, task after task, until the sand in the hourglass runs out—or until it has been so long since you considered what you really wanted that you can no longer remember what it was.

DO THE OPPOSITE

All right. Here's the wink at last. You and I both know that you don't really aspire to the goals set out in this chapter. You've explored the valleys of depression enough. You're looking for the mountaintops instead. What might the upward path look like?

Ordinarily, a densely packed and unfailingly social restaurant might draw us in. When we are sad or depressed, however, we will feel drawn to our own home, where we can simply thaw out some leftovers and be left in peace. Normally the prospect of a run by the ocean might seem idyllic. When we are overtaken with ennui, such a pursuit may only seem pointless and tiring. The resulting choices—inactivity, isolation, procrastination—often serve only to magnify the intensity of the negative state.

This phenomenon can be so pronounced that I offer it as a general principle to any client suffering from misery. When you are feeling down, the majority of temptations you experience will lead you even lower.

It is as though our emotions mutiny and jump ship, switching their allegiance to our worst enemy: despair. By following the siren song of their exhortations ("Call in sick and close the curtains, you'll feel better!"), we will only erode our mood further.

Instead, when our mood darkens we need to treat our instincts with suspicion. Usually we will experience relief only when we learn to act against our temptations, often engaging in what psychologist Marsha Linehan (developer of dialectical behavior therapy) calls Opposite Action. We feel tempted to withdraw, and so we approach instead. We feel exhausted, but we use this as our cue to get more exercise. Itching to defend ourselves by attacking others, we instead cultivate compassion. Agitated and antsy, we take ten minutes to sit quietly and meditate.

We notice the impulse, know that it leads downward, and turn right rather than left.

Taking Action

Perhaps, when life deals you a series of blows, you typically find yourself gorging on junk food—which serves only to make you feel ill and bloated. The temptation has been there in the past and will probably return next time as well. Rather than simply hoping that this doesn't happen, what could you do to intervene when it does?

You can monitor your external stresses—the elements of life that are beyond your control—and make a point of taking note when they come at you too hard or too quickly. Knowing your attraction to junk food at such times, you could increase your vigilance for impulse purchases at the grocery store, making more of a point of keeping to your shopping list. You could buy snack food that will do you less harm or that you do not find quite so tempting. You could also give yourself permission to go out for fast food now and then—but perhaps not quite as often as your impulses might dictate.

In many cases, this will involve putting the brakes on the downhill slide. But you can also push yourself to turn around and move toward a happier state instead.

For each of your most prominent downward temptations, develop a plan to arrest the slide and turn in the opposite direction. Do not attempt to put these plans into effect all at once. Spreading your efforts across too many fronts is itself a trap. Work on no more than two or three tendencies at a time. When they become a bit easier (no one ever fully masters or erases them), take on new ones.

When you know there are temptations that are simply too powerful to resist, simply acknowledge the choice point that you are sliding past. Do so in an accepting manner. It is a choice. By becoming increasingly aware of the fork in the road, you lay the groundwork for someday taking the other path.

Dr. Rich's Depression Remedy: Guided Imagery

Guided imagery is a manly mental journey that trains your mind's eye to zero in on hope, strength, and small wins. Try closing your eyes and picturing yourself standing in a cool mountain stream. Or, better yet, grab a fly rod and actually do it. Either way, let the calming effects wash over you.

Want more manly tips on Depression? Explore the Gentlemental Health card on **ManTherapy.org**.

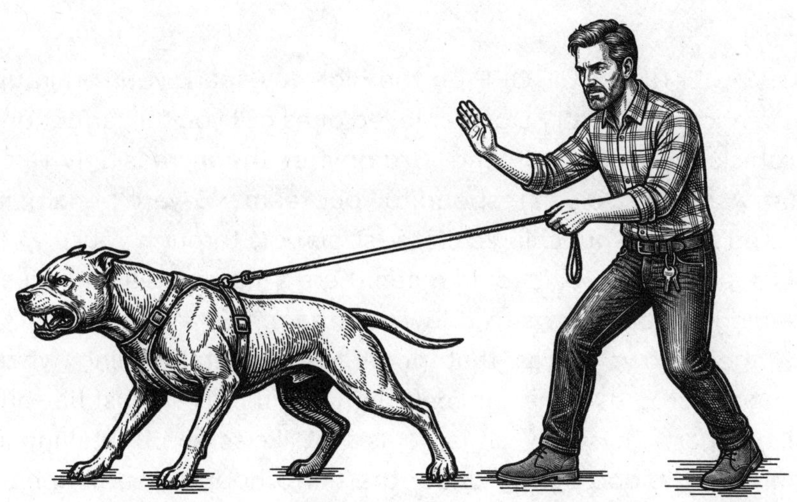

ANGER

TRAINING YOUR TEMPER

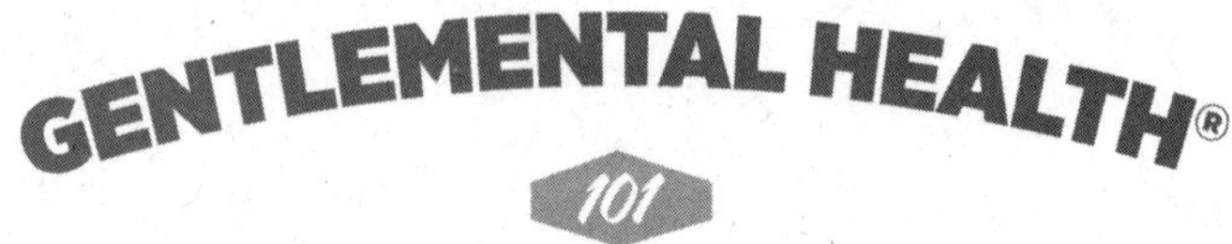

DOES GETTING CUT OFF on the highway spark your brain up like a nuclear reactor? Do your loved ones call you fun, affectionate nicknames like Hothead, Grumpy, or the increasingly relevant: Asshole? Do you respond to your team's 15-yard penalty in the red zone by punching a crater-sized hole through your TV? If this sounds like you, it could mean there's more at play than just needing effective ways to "blow off steam."

Anger shows up as that pedal-to-the-metal feeling when someone crosses a line, life feels unfair, or things are just flat-out falling apart. Physically, anger feels a lot like screws tightening in your chest, blood boiling under the skin, choppy breathing patterns, and fists clenched as if ready for a fight. Mentally and emotionally, anger shows up as violent impulses, loss of emotional control, inability to accept reality, erratic tendencies, and even suicidal ideation. Anger also frequently hides deeper-rooted issues like depression, anxiety, trauma, or shame.

When it comes to anger, the most important question to ask yourself is, "Does it control me or do I control it?" As noted, plenty of things set us off, make us defensive, or want to punch back. When men are raised to think that they can't be sad, hurt, or scared, the only acceptable emotion left in those moments is anger. However, if anger gets a vice grip on us, it can lead to destructive outcomes.

The good news is that it is possible to get a hold on anger. There are effective methods for addressing it—building in a "cool down" period when anger rises, affirming yourself when feeling slighted, repeating mantras when feeling threatened, avoiding common triggers, or talking to a therapist—to make sure that you can keep cool when your internal thermometer rises.

While acting on that angry impulse may make you feel better in the short term, when it comes to anger, the long-term downsides often outweigh the release you feel in the moment. If you can learn how to train your temper and remain in control of your emotions, you can direct that energy toward a more focused, measured, and intentional outcome. Learning how to harness the powerful surge of aggression can then become your hidden superpower.

For more insights on turning a kryptonite into a strength, let's check in with a couple of experts— Matthew McKay and Peter D. Rogers—to start manhandling anger.

WHY DO GUYS GET SO ANGRY?

MATTHEW MCKAY, PHD, AND PETER D. ROGERS, PHD

As psychologists with a combined fifty-two years in practice, we've come to some conclusions about the problem of anger:

- For most people, chronic anger covers incredible pain. And while anger often feels like a release at the moment, it inevitably makes the underlying pain worse.

- Of those people who suffered the greatest damage in childhood, most were harmed by repeated exposure to anger. The majority of chronically angry people were also damaged by anger as children.

- People struggling with chronic anger suffer long-term consequences in both work and personal relationships. They tend to feel more alone, more disappointed by life, and less nourished by their relationships.

- The greatest predictor of satisfaction in marriage is how people learn to handle conflict and anger.

- Anger is a learned response, and the anger response can be unlearned with commitment and effort.

Anger is ubiquitous in our society, from road rage to the soaring incidence of child physical abuse. Everyone is touched by it. Over the years, and tens of thousands of hours of therapy, we have seen what it costs our clients—both those who struggle with overwhelming bouts of anger, and those who are its victims. The regret, the loss, the hurt and fear leave deep scars on everyone.

Where Is It Really Coming From?

Anger isn't always about the current annoyance—this nitwit who can't take a message, or the person who cut in front of you at the toll plaza. Often the roots of anger can be traced back to earlier times when you were hurt, abused, or neglected in your family of origin. The pain was something you carried, year after year. It may have left scars so that now it's hard to feel safe or loved or truly worthy. Sometimes it doesn't take much of a provocation to trigger those feelings of being unloved, unworthy, or unsafe—and the anger rises up right alongside that old pain.

From the very start, it's important to get one thing straight. You aren't to blame because you struggle with anger. You are not a bad person because you've forgotten—perhaps repeatedly—all your resolutions to be cool and calm. Rather, you are a person in pain. Whether the pain is occasional or chronic, when it hits, it feels overwhelming. It's a wave that drives you into a state of mind where nothing matters but expressing what you feel. You shout it out. No matter who gets hurt or whatever the consequences.

Anger is a way of coping. It helps, temporarily, to overcome the hurt and helplessness. For a moment you feel back in control, and that's exactly why anger is so hard to manage. If you try to put a cork in your anger, you may feel acutely the pain that triggered it.

So now is the time to stop kicking yourself. It doesn't help. In fact, blaming yourself for your anger simply creates more pain—bad, unworthy feelings—and the pain triggers more anger. It's a self-perpetuating cycle. If you're going to get off this merry-go-round, you'll need another way to view your anger problem. Your anger is:

- A response you learned early in life to cope with pain.

- A way, however temporary, to overcome feelings of help-lessness and lack of control.

- A habit that, up till now, you've lacked the tools to break.

Acquiring new anger management tools will take time, probably two to four months. That's the bad news. But the good news is that you can learn them and, in doing so, change your life. They're right here—keep reading, and keep doing the exercises. And there's more good news. While it will take time to learn your new anger management skills, there's something you can do about your anger right now—today.

ACTIVITY
Personal Costs of Anger

In the space of a private journal, write brief descriptions of how anger has affected you in each area. Put an asterisk by any num-bered item that feels like a crucial reason for you to learn more about anger management.

1. How anger has affected my work relationships (include jobs lost or jeopardized)

2. How anger has affected the relationships to my family of origin (including parents, siblings, and extended family)

3. How anger has affected my marriage or intimate/romantic relationships

4. How anger has affected my children

5. How anger has affected my friendships (including lost friends and strained relationships)

6. How my anger has harmed people who aren't family or friends (including the names of all the people my anger has hurt—on a separate sheet if necessary)

7. How my anger has affected my health and physical well-being (including stress-related illnesses/problems and physical discomfort from anger reactions)

8. How anger has endangered me (including reckless driving, physical fights, hurting myself by hitting things, legal problems, etc.)

9. How anger has affected me financially (include bad decisions made in anger as well as material things broken or damaged)

10. How anger has affected me spiritually (including bad behavior that goes against my personal code of ethics or sense of right and wrong)

With all the negatives associated with anger, why are you still blowing up? Why does anger remain such a powerful force in your life? Why, even when you resolve to control it, does your anger still flare up? In this chapter you'll find answers to these questions. A good place to start is understanding the five short-term payoffs that anger can provide.

Anger Payoffs

Anger reduces stress. Stress can come from a lot of sources—worry, frustration, unmet needs, physical pain or discomfort, rushing against deadlines, and so on. You don't need this book to tell you about your stress. What's important is the link between stress and anger. Stress creates physiological arousal—tension. The greater the stress, and the number of stressors, the more unpleasant is the arousal you feel.

Anger discharges arousal, but only temporarily. Right after a blowup, people often feel oddly relaxed, like a weight has been lifted off their shoulders. It seems like they can breathe again. Even though these effects are brief, and tension soon returns, the anger discharge can be highly reinforcing. You get a break from everything that frustrates and overwhelms you.

But there's a downside to using anger for stress reduction. The stress comes back with a vengeance. Studies show that anger creates more anger. Blowing up makes it more likely that you'll blow up again soon. Each time you indulge in anger to cope with stress, the next outburst becomes that much easier and stronger—and harder to control.

Not only does your anger get worse, but so does the anger of those around you. They get hurt and defensive. They counterattack. And they harden, becoming less and less concerned about your needs and feelings.

Short-term, then, anger is a good strategy for discharging

stress arousal. But it tends to boomerang. Later, you pay dearly in the coin of broken relationships.

Anger hides emotional pain. Anger is a good defense against fear, loss, guilt, shame, and feelings of rejection or failure. It puts a tight lid on painful emotions, locking most of the feelings out of awareness. Growing up in dysfunctional families, we watch Dad push away his shame with rage. Or Mom cope with her depression by yelling at the kids. We learn that we can stop virtually any painful feeling if we can just get mad enough.

But once again, the short-term payoff has long-term consequences. First of all, you don't let yourself experience feelings that may be important signals, offering guidance for what you need to do or stop doing in your life. Maybe there's a good reason you feel guilt, and you need to face it and do something about it. Maybe you need to face your depression, taking responsibility to make key changes in your life.

The second problem with using anger to defend against your feelings is that the feelings often get worse over time. You're not only guilty for some past failure—now you feel guilty for the new damage your anger has done. Or the depression worsens because your anger is turning people off and isolating you. Now you have to crank up your anger even more to block these higher levels of guilt or sadness.

The third problem with using anger as a defense is that it becomes habitual. The anger reflex seems to go off at the slightest criticism or hurt, or the slightest anxiety. Say you're a little worried while trying to figure out the bills. Boom! It's a lot easier to blow up because your partner bought a sixty-dollar espresso maker than to feel uncertainty about your finances.

Anger gets your attention. Sometimes it seems that no one listens to you unless you're yelling. Anger does grab people's attention. They get alarmed and sometimes they'll try to placate you. But once again, the immediate payoff has long-term outcomes that hurt you. First, a certain percentage of people don't respond to anger with attentive listening. They get immediately defensive and tune you out. They start avoiding you or, worse, they hold it against you. The problem is that you've chosen a strategy that makes some people sit up and listen, and some people run.

The second problem with using anger to get attention is that the people who responded initially get inured and hardened over time. They stop being alarmed by your anger and start being disgusted by it. Instead of listening, they resent you and shut down.

Anger may be used for punishment and revenge. Someone really lets you down. They screw up because they're lazy or stupid or don't care about you. Inside is this huge wave of rage. You want to punish them and teach them a lesson. You want them to feel as much pain as you do. God, it feels good. This righteousness, this will to harm, is so powerful that it's all you care about. You hunger for the opportunity to get back at them—whether it's a screamed insult or a carefully planned revenge.

The trouble is, each time you act on these impulses, you make enemies, and the enemies often end up being the people you love and need most. Naturally, your enemies want to punish you. The world becomes a stage for bitter struggles, where old hurts and grudges push each of you to new excesses of rage and aggression.

Anger can help you change others. In dysfunctional families, we learn to use anger to extort things from others. We coerce them with blowups, or the fear of blowups, into complying with our demands. It's tempting to use anger as a club because, at least in the short term, people often give you what you want.

In the long run, of course, they turn off and turn away from you. They resent being controlled by fear. But worst of all is what it does to you. Using your anger to change others leaves you feeling helpless. When you're in pain, when something hurts, it always seems like the other person has to fix it. You feel powerless to overcome the problem yourself. And all you know how to do is try to coerce the other person into corrective action.

By placing the responsibility to change a painful situation

outside yourself, you are starting down the royal slippery slope toward helplessness and depression. You're leaving others in charge of your pain and your life.

How You Get Angry

Anger is a two-step process. It starts with the experience of pain. The pain can be physical or emotional—it could be a stomach-ache or fatigue, feelings of rejection or loss. The pain can be something that frustrates your needs or threatens your safety. The particular kind of pain doesn't matter. What's important is that the pain by definition is unpleasant and makes you want to put an end to it. The second component of the anger response is trigger thoughts. These are interpretations, assumptions, and evaluations of a situation that make you feel victimized and deliberately harmed by others. Trigger thoughts blame and con-demn others for the painful experience you've suffered.

You might think of emotional or physical pain as the fuel of anger. It's like a can of gasoline, and your trigger thoughts are the match. Either of the anger components alone is harmless. Pain by itself doesn't ignite rage, and trigger thoughts without pain are like a match without fuel.

Pain plus trigger thoughts equals anger. It's a simple formula. Imagine that you have a headache and your fourteen-year-old starts nagging you about going to a party that will involve drink-ing. She keeps pushing, and your head keeps pounding. Her pressure and the pain in your head aren't enough to get angry. You need a match—a trigger thought that says she's an inconsid-erate kid who doesn't give a damn about how tired you are. Now the anger catches fire. You're hurting, and you have someone to blame. You've decided who's responsible for your pain. The next words out of your mouth are loud and attacking. Your daughter stares at you like you just went nuts, but in reality it was a simple matter of putting the fuel and match together.

Once you get angry, trigger thoughts can also make it worse. They can escalate your upset by continually painting the other person as bad and wrong and deliberately out to harm you. Each new trigger thought pushes your anger a notch higher, until you end up saying and doing very damaging things. Pain begets trigger thoughts, which beget anger, more trigger thoughts, more anger, and so on. Your thoughts and angry feelings become a self-perpetuating feedback loop.

Here are several important questions you should consider (we recommend tracking anger episodes to find patterns):

- What types of stresses or pain typically foreshadow high anger episodes? Are any of these stresses preventable? Could they be calmed or coped with in ways other than anger?

- What types of provocative situations are typically associated with high anger episodes? Is there a common theme or dynamic to high anger situations?

- What category of trigger thought most angers you (i.e., feeling treated unjustly, not being cared about, being ignored, blaming others, negative labels like "stupid" or "selfish," assuming ill will, etc.)?

- Do you behave differently in response to moderate anger as opposed to high anger experiences? How would you like to change the way you express your anger?

- Are the outcomes more negative for high as opposed to moderate anger experiences?

- Are the outcomes from your anger experiences more often positive or negative? If negative, are the outcomes affecting you temporarily or also in the long term?

- Is your anger affecting others in ways that concern you?

- Are there specific trigger thoughts or trigger thought themes that seem to generate the most negative outcomes?

- Are there particular behaviors that seem to trigger more negative outcomes, either for yourself or others?

It's good to start asking them now, because careful observation of your anger helps to build motivation to complete an anger control program.

ACTIVITY
Twenty-Four-Hour Commitment to Act Calm

Notice it isn't a commitment to be calm, just to act that way. Effective anger management starts with a specific, time-limited decision. You need to commit to yourself and to key people in your life that you are going to behave in a calm, nonaggressive way. Not forever. That's impossible; no one could promise such a thing. Not even for a week. That's far too long, given how strong and habitual your anger response might be. Your commitment is just for a single twenty-four-hour day.

Here's how you make it work:

1. **Tell people.** Share with every significant person in your life that you are absolutely committed to behaving in a calm way between __________ and __________ . Explain that this means you won't shout at, swear at, hit, blame, attack, or denigrate anyone. Absolutely. No exceptions or excuses. Let them know that you're going to be vigilant and on

guard for aggressive behavior throughout the designated time period.

2. **Ask for help.** There's a good chance—especially if you experience frequent, unpredictable anger—that this won't be easy. So you need real help, not just people's good wishes. Give family and friends a nonverbal signal they can use to let you know if you're looking or sounding angry. Something like a referee's time-out sign, or the gesture an umpire uses when a player slides in safe, or just a slowly descending hand that means "relax, calm down." Whatever signal you want to use, write it down and tell people how it works.

3. **Prepare yourself in advance,** that whenever you see the signal you will stop talking until you can once again appear calm. Remember, you don't have to be calm, just act calm.

4. **Sign a contract.** Have one close person sign as witness to the contract.

5. **See the benefit.** What's the number-one thing you want to achieve through anger management? A better relationship with your spouse, your kids, your friends? A chance to heal old wounds with your family? A better shot at rewards and promotions at work? A renewed feeling of pride and self-worth? An end to dangerous or costly behavior? Whatever is your biggest and best reason for acting calm.

6. **Plan for provocations.** Assume that during the twenty-four hours, things will happen to upset you. A few of them you can probably even anticipate.

To face these or similar anger triggers, you'll need a few simple strategies.

What to Do When You Get Angry

1. First, and most important, stop. Don't do or say anything. Don't act on the angry feelings. This is just an emotion. It's a strong one, but you can feel it without turning it into behavior.

2. Try to step back from the feeling and label it. Notice its strength: be aware of how it pushes you toward action. Accept it. There's nothing inherently wrong with anger. It's just a signal that you're in pain. The only problem is when you act on anger to hurt others or yourself.

3. Don't push the feeling away, but don't try to hold onto it either. It will come like a wave—building, cresting, then slowly receding. Let it come, and then let it go. Watch how it grows and diminishes, as if you were a scientist observing some interesting phenomenon. Take care not to do anything to amplify your anger. Don't dwell on the unfairness of the situation.

4. Don't review past failings of the offending individual. Don't rehearse in your mind the events leading to your anger. Just notice and accept the feeling, watching as it gradually diminishes.

ACT THE OPPOSITE

One of the quickest ways to change a painful feeling is to act the opposite. During your twenty-four-hour commitment to calm behavior, anger can be a signal to put a very different face on your emotions.

- Smile instead of frown. The very act of smiling when angry tends to diminish the strength of your upset feelings.

- Speak softly rather than loudly. Go overboard on this. Make your voice lower and gentler than usual; try to make it soothing.

- Relax instead of tighten. Let your arms hang loose. Take a breath. Lean against something in a casual way or sit with your legs crossed comfortably. Look calm, even if you don't feel it.

- Disengage rather than attack. You may want to get right in the other person's face. You may want to shake them—emotionally if not physically. Instead, look or walk away. Make no comment about the provoking situation. Save it for another time. You'll only blow up if you try to deal with this now.

- Empathize rather than judge. Say something mildly supportive, such as, "This is a difficult situation for you," or "I can see why you're concerned (upset, overwhelmed, dismayed, etc.)." It's okay if you don't feel supportive and the words seem phony. You can have a strong desire to take a two-by-four to the other person. But just behave as if you can appreciate their point of view. "You rammed the car into the garage door? (gritting your teeth) When you're rushed, it's easy to get rattled." "You got a D+ on your math test? (rapidly growing knot in your stomach) You've been distracted, I think, but we can get back on track."

BEYOND THE FIRST TWENTY-FOUR HOURS

When you've gotten through the first twenty-four-hours, you have a choice. Make additional twenty-four-hour commitments or monitor your anger. In either case, start working to build your new anger management skills.

Notice the word "working" in the last sentence. Simply reading this book isn't enough. It will take a real effort to change such a powerful response habit. And you'll need to practice your new skills every day. It's going to take time and energy, but the benefits you'll achieve by changing your angry behavior will be more than worth it.

RECOGNIZING TRIGGER THOUGHTS

You can always tell an anger-triggering thought by how it frames reality. Here are the basic components of most trigger thoughts:

- The perception that you've been harmed and victimized.

- The belief that the provoking person harmed you deliberately.

- The belief that the provoking person was wrong and bad to harm you, and should have behaved differently.

Let's examine some typical trigger thoughts and see how these three elements can be separated out:

"WHY DO I HAVE TO COME HOME FROM WORK EXHAUSTED AND SHOP AND CLEAN AND COOK AND GET ZERO HELP?"

Harm: Overwork, exhaustion
Done Deliberately: Implication that the provoking person chooses not to help, thus contributing to the exhaustion.
And Wrong: Implication that giving zero help is unjust and unfair.

"IT'S A STUPID WAY TO OPERATE A CAR, AND I'VE SAID IT A HUNDRED TIMES—YOU DON'T KEEP RIDING THE BRAKES BECAUSE IT WEARS THEM OUT."

Harm: Cost of a brake job; not being listened to.

Done Deliberately: Implication that if the provoking person thought a little more, or made a reasonable effort, he or she could remember to use the brakes properly.

And Wrong: Implies that riding the brakes is poor driving technique, and not heeding appropriate warnings is either lazy or careless.

"SHE'S DOING THIS TO UPSET ME (CHILD JUMPING ON THE SOFA FOLLOWING AN ANGRY EXCHANGE REGARDING STAYING AT THE TABLE UNTIL BREAKFAST IS EATEN)."

Harm: Noise, dirt on sofa, not being listened to.

Done Deliberately: Implies the child is choosing obnoxious behavior out of a need for revenge.

And Wrong: Implies child is being manipulative and disobedient.

All trigger thoughts assert that you've been harmed, deliberately and wrongly. But there's one more implication: Not only did the provoking person cause your pain, but they ought to change so the pain can stop. They are both responsible for the harm and required to fix it.

The problem with this thinking is that it leaves you feeling very helpless. The pain you experience is out of your control. Someone did it to you, and you won't feel better until they see the light and change their behavior. But, as you already know, people rarely change. They keep behaving in habitual ways. They do what's rewarding to them, what makes them feel good. Your anger may distress them briefly, but usually they quickly return to their old patterns. The whole time you're angry, waiting for them to change, you remain stuck. You keep hurting, and the problem feels beyond your control.

This feeling of angry helplessness starts a vicious cycle: You're hurt, the provoking person should fix it but doesn't, and you feel stuck and unable to escape the pain. The feeling of helplessness makes you feel even worse, even more angry, even more frustrated that the provoking person won't change.

Breaking the cycle requires that you take responsibility for changing what's painful, and not wait for the other person to do it. For example, imagine that you have a friend who's chronically late for lunch dates. Over and over you find yourself fuming in a restaurant. Of course, you can lambaste your friend each time you find yourself stuck waiting; you can complain about the thoughtlessness and disregard for your time. However, if you take responsibility for your own pain, you might:

- always remember to bring a book and schedule extra time, or

- never meet in a restaurant, or

- always include others so you'll have someone to talk to while you wait, or

- pick your friend up at home.

When you take responsibility, both anger and helplessness melt away. You're suddenly free to solve the problem. Instead of always asking the question, "Who's responsible for my pain?" you ask instead, "What can I do about it?"

Here are three coping mantras that can help you stay focused on taking responsibility:

- I am responsible for what happens between us.

- No point in blaming. I'll try a new strategy for taking care of myself.

- What can I do about this?

We know that how you think about things determines to a large degree what you experience, and this is particularly true of anger. For now, however, it's only necessary to understand that coping thoughts are different ways of conceptualizing or reframing a situation in order to help you to better manage your anger.

BLAMING

This is the most self-destructive and damaging anger distortion. The mistaken belief that underlies blaming is that other people are doing bad things to you, usually on purpose—and they aren't going to get away with it. It's true that blaming other people can make you feel better sometimes, but it leaves you feeling helpless as well. By blaming others, you are giving up the power to change the situation that is causing you pain. You keep waiting for them to change their behavior. But, of course, they never do. This can cause you to be judgmental and vindictive, lashing out angrily. The other person then responds by pulling back or counterattacking. Now you've got two problems, the original situation and the mess you've made with your angry reaction.

EXAMPLES OF BLAMING

- I could really enjoy this vacation if it weren't for your constant complaining and always finding fault with things.

- If you really cared about me, you would have helped me with the résumé, and then I would have gotten that job.

- You always ask me to give you a ride and then take all day to get dressed, so I'll be late for my meeting.

It's useful to remember that people are mostly doing the best they can. Everyone (including you) tends to behave in ways that will meet their own needs. The people you're blaming are most likely just doing what they can to take care of themselves as best they know how.

When you use a blaming strategy, your entire focus is on trying to change the other person. What's easy to forget is that you're not stuck. You can make different choices. Remember that you have some options to change the situation—it doesn't all depend on the other person. The key to dealing with self-defeating blaming is to develop a new coping strategy. This requires you to take responsibility and make your own plan to change the situation, or to figure out a different way of responding to it. Forget the other person—they're not going to do anything different. Therefore, your plan shouldn't require any cooperation whatsoever from the person you blame.

COPING THOUGHTS TO REPLACE BLAMING

- I know that blaming makes me feel helpless, so what can I do to change the situation and make myself feel better?

- I can make a plan to take care of myself in this situation.

- I don't like what he's doing, but I know that he's just trying to take care of himself.

- I'm hurt and disappointed, but I believe that she's doing the best she can.

- I'm not helpless, and I can take care of myself in this situation.

- They're doing what they need to do, so I'll just have to do what I need to do.

INFLAMMATORY GLOBAL LABELING

This anger distortion involves making sweeping, often inflammatory, negative judgments about people whose behavior you don't like. However, instead of focusing on the behavior, the label tends to paint the person as being totally wrong, bad, and worthless. This is accomplished by one-word epithets like "loser," "asshole," "jerk," "retard," "bitch," "bastard," or "schmuck." Global labels tend to fuel your anger by turning the person whose behavior you don't like into a worthless object. And, of course the labels are always false and misleading because they reduce the whole person to a single characteristic.

EXAMPLES OF INFLAMMATORY GLOBAL LABELING

- My girlfriend is a total bitch.

- That driver who just cut me off is a complete asshole.

- What a jerk. He doesn't know anything.

- That bastard deserves to be drawn and quartered for what he did to me.

- Look at that wimpy tennis serve—he's a real loser.

The best way to combat a tendency toward global labeling is to be specific. Focus on the annoying behavior and describe it with precision. What happened? When did it happen? How often? How did it affect you or others? Notice that this does not involve making judgments about the other person or making derogatory comments about his/her personality or parentage.

COPING THOUGHTS TO REPLACE INFLAMMATORY GLOBAL LABELING

- Why am I swearing? I feel frustrated, and things aren't going the way I would like. But I can cope with the situation.

- It's nothing more than a problem. I don't have to make her the wicked witch.

- What is really bothering me? Stick to the facts.

- He's not a jerk, just someone who wasn't properly trained to do his job.

MISATTRIBUTIONS

This is all about jumping to conclusions and mind reading. When you find yourself feeling hurt or annoyed by other people's behavior, the simplest thing is to imagine that they did it on purpose. Rather than thinking about all the other reasons for why things might have happened as they did, you assume that you know the person's "real" motives. You focus on a single explanation. They were deliberately trying to be mean to you and cause you upset.

It's easy to guess at other people's motives. But if you've ever taken the trouble to check out your assumptions, you've no doubt discovered how often you were partly or completely mistaken. Sometimes misattributions can cause real problems, such as when you angrily act on your mistaken assumptions, only to find out later that the true situation was entirely different from what you imagined.

EXAMPLES OF MISATTRIBUTIONS

- He acted like he just wanted to correct my grammar, but he was really trying to make me look stupid.

- I know she was just doing that to embarrass me in front of everyone.

- What a dumb assignment. He's really out to get me.

- The only reason she's late is just to piss me off.

The best way to avoid misattributions is to pay attention and catch yourself making the assumptions. Then, if possible, check it out with the person directly or gather some relevant facts. If you're reluctant to directly check out your assumptions, at least keep an open mind to other possibilities. Consider asking someone you trust what they make of a certain situation, to get another point of view.

Sometimes your interpretations of other people's behavior might actually be correct. However, there are usually many other reasons or explanations for people's actions—things that might surprise you. Your anger may be way out of line or disproportionate to the situation. A good way to work on misattribution is to get into the habit of developing alternative explanations for other people's behavior. Really brainstorm: Try to think of as many different scenarios as you can, and think of your original assumption as just one of many possible explanations of how other people act.

COPING THOUGHTS TO REPLACE MISATTRIBUTIONS

- That's one possibility, but there are probably other reasons for her behavior.

- Stop trying to second-guess other people's motives.

- Getting angry won't help me figure out what's really going on. I need more facts.

- My assumption may not be accurate—I'd better check it out.

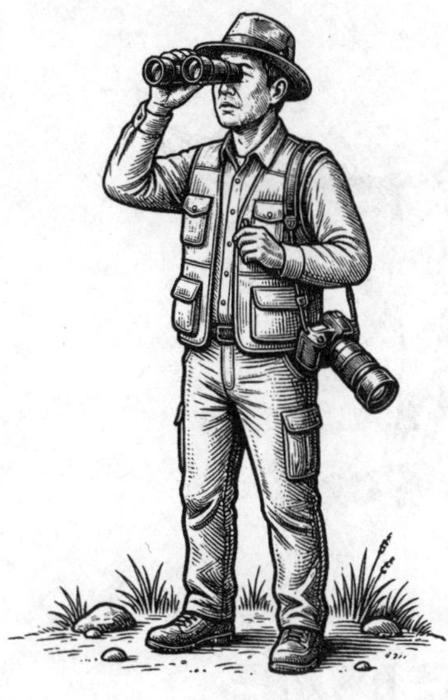

Dr. Rich's Anger Remedy: Bird Watching

Anger got you wrenched? A great way to train your temper is finding easy ways to get out of your head and help those internal gears grind to a halt. Turns out there's something oddly relaxing about watching our tiny feathered friends go bananas over a bit of birdseed.

Want more manly tips on Anger? Explore the Gentlemental Health card on **ManTherapy.org**.

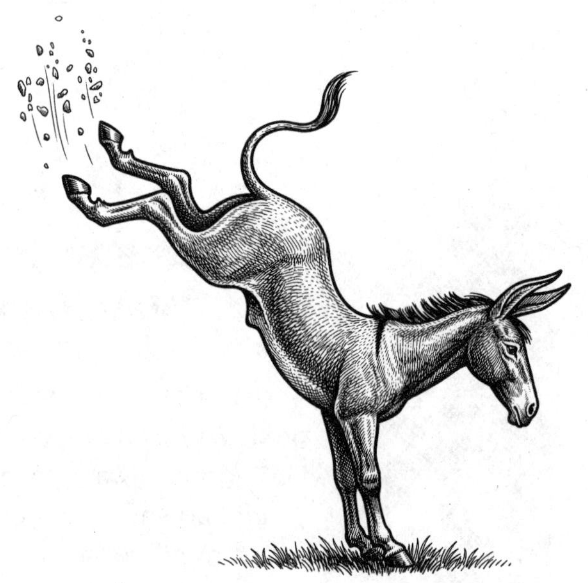

IMPULSIVE BEHAVIOR AND ADDICTION

KICK THE HABIT BEFORE IT KICKS YOUR ASS

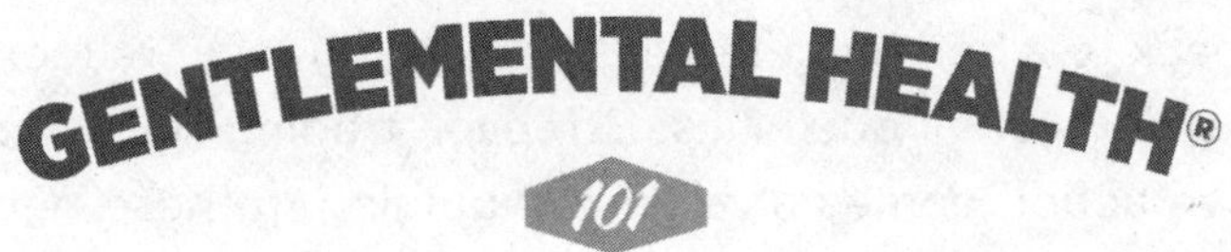

THERE'S NO BEATING AROUND THE BUSH: addiction is a son-of-a-gun. As soon as you think you've pinned it, it'll flip you six ways from Sunday and lock you in a full nelson. The road to addiction starts at the intersection of impulsivity and curiosity. After being on the wagon for months, you start wondering if a sip of beer is really so bad, and next thing you know that seemingly harmless curiosity pushes you off the wagon.

Impulse and addiction are inextricably linked because they share the same brain circuitry. Impulsive behavior and addiction can both:

- **Weaken your regulatory system.** The part of your brain that oversees self-control decreases, meaning you are less likely to override your own impulses, which can lead to addictive behavior.

- **Increase the desire for immediate gratification.** Impulse and addiction spur an overactive, dopamine-fueled reward system, which means, like a little brat in a toy store, you want what you want when you want it.

- **Create an imbalance in threat detection.** Not only do you get stuck in harmful behavior patterns, you also lose the ability to regulate whether or not you're putting yourself in danger.

Newsflash: it's called impulsive behavior because we find ourselves doing something without thinking about the action or its consequences. We also create our own reasons for impulsively going back to a bad habit because of the urgency we feel based on the story we tell ourselves. However, trading self-control for impulsive action comes at a cost. Indulging in these behaviors can lead to increased anxiety, depression, intrusive thoughts, disrupted sleep, shame spirals, and deterioration in overall health. Not to mention, following those impulses can eventually saddle you with an addiction.

Let's be clear, these behaviors are not confined to excessive drinking, drug use, and gambling. Men can get hooked on just about anything: porn, gaming, social media, adrenaline, food, shopping, exercise, work, etc. These indulgences don't always look the same, but they can overlap or be substitutes for each other.

As with any pattern, recognizing it can spur action to address it. It can start simply, like knowing your triggers and creating a plan to tackle them. You can try urge surfing: let impulses rise, recognize them for what they are—a fleeting pull to do something harmful—and let them fade. If you feel pinned down by addiction, you can always seek professional help in the form of therapy or support groups.

Remember, when you're addicted, you're surrendering control. So, let's learn from a pro's pro, Michael Barnett, on how we can get those behaviors in checkmate.

ADDICTIVE BEHAVIORS

MICHAEL BARNETT, LPCC

Despite more than one hundred years of scientific research, addiction has become to the field of behavioral health what the common cold is to the field of medicine: ubiquitous. It can affect anyone and occur at any time. Even with profound medical advances capable of mapping the impact of addiction on the brain in exquisite detail, addiction has escalated exponentially. In this very moment, you are among thousands of people earnestly seeking relief who have been unable to find a way out.

The reality is that we can never effectively overcome our addictive behaviors if we can't identify and understand its root cause. We know all too well that addiction is a powerful (and reliable) way to avoid and numb emotion. However, truth be told, *none of us* learned to avoid feeling our feelings randomly—we needed to keep them at bay for very good reasons, which we will get to later. Plain and simple, emotional pain without dependable people to offer reassurance and support means one must find another source of relief. For so many of us, drugs, gambling, or alcohol become that option. Substances, and addictive activities, can offer temporary relief (at best) from emotional pain. However, in time, as you know all too well, addiction eventually takes on a life of its own. Alternatively, when life's road gets rocky, when we know in our bones that there are people to whom we can turn who care about us, we are infinitely stronger, more resilient, and safe.

The Common Misconception About Addiction

The addiction treatment field—as well as the experts, counselors, and leaders within it—has not come to a conclusive perspective about the causes of addiction nor how to effectively treat it (Alexander 2008). Most of the leading opinions regarding the causes of addiction include a degree of stigma and judgment about a person's character or capability. An inherently shaming thread runs through most of our contemporary perspectives about addiction, leaving us feeling bad about ourselves. The shocking paradox is that the very protocols and processes that were designed to help break the chains of addiction have often been a source of shame and additional distress, which ironically further activates the need to self-medicate with substances (Finberg 2015).

For the record, we don't have character defects. We are not broken, diseased, lowly, or too weak to contend with chemicals and urges. We are human beings who have not always been dealt the easiest hand of cards. Therefore, we need a more complete and humane definition of addiction if we are to grow and heal in such a way that we can release the hold of addiction once and for all.

When we cast stigmas and misconceptions aside, we can look more compassionately at addiction and ourselves. Here is a description I've found eliminates shame and gets to the truth: *Addictive processes help us cope with often-unbearable emotional suffering and distress when the support and care of dependable others is simply not an option.*

This revised understanding is both human and non-pathologizing. It acknowledges that life is challenging, that no one gets out unscathed. It views addiction for what it is: functional. Addiction serves a meaningful purpose: it helps us cope with emotional and personal suffering that, for some of us, is unbearable (Maté 2007).

This new perspective offers hope and possibility. It provides a guide for creating healthy alternatives to lighten our load and helps prop us up when the going gets tough.

The bumps, bruises, and hardships of life are bearable only if we have the safe haven of community and caring others to lean into when the going gets tough. Although a sense of belonging within a community should be a birthright, it is far from a given. Therefore, I want you to know that whatever feels addictive to you is not your fault. However, changing your relationship with the addictive processes that have compromised your life *is your responsibility*.

The good news is that successfully accomplishing this is truly within your reach.

Change Is Not Only Possible, It's Probable!

It may feel disorienting to discover that there is a vast body of epidemiological research (Hasin et al. 2007) revealing that the majority of people who struggle with addictive processes stop using on their own accord, without any form of professional intervention whatsoever. But it's true!

Natural recovery is an organic life process that leads to recovery without formal treatment or self-help groups. It typically involves struggling with strong feelings that one's using is incongruent with the kind of person they want to be—that is, discordant with their own values, aspirations, and life goals (Heyman 2009). Usually, natural recovery happens over a period of several years of attempting to stop but not yet achieving recovery goals...until one day the transformation of one's relationship to addiction is successful.

Not knowing that most people recover naturally from addictive processes can leave you feeling doomed to having a very low ceiling on your life and personal aspirations. Research shows that 75 percent of people struggling with addictive behaviors successfully change their relationship to using substances and behaviors either through abstinence or harm reduction (Blanco et al. 2011). When viewed through this lens, changing your relationship to your addiction becomes a genuine possibility—maybe more so than you have ever considered.

It is absolutely essential that you understand that you too are destined for recovery. There really is light at the end of the tunnel!

ACTIVITY
Anchoring Success Inside of Yourself

STEP 1: The Habit You Broke

Think of a simple nagging habit that you have struggled with that you don't do anymore. Perhaps it was biting your fingernails, not exercising regularly, eating more then you were comfortable with, isolating and not socializing as much as you might like, procrastinating...the list goes on. Identify a time when you decided to shift gears and did so successfully by responding to these prompts in a journal or notebook.

The habit that I broke:

What I did to successfully accomplish it:

How I felt as a result of quitting successfully:

STEP 2: Visualizing Success

Close your eyes and prepare as you normally would for a visualization practice. Remembering your success in stopping a nagging habit, exclusively focus on the feelings you just wrote down as a result of your success. If your mind drifts elsewhere, gently bring it back to those successful feelings inside. Stay with them for a minute or two. Notice where they live inside of your body. What does the sensation in your body feel like? Tingly, warm, calm? Gently breathe into these feelings of success as you allow yourself to reconnect with them and internalize them. We want to "grow" the experience of these feelings until they become a familiar staple of your daily life. Stay with these sensations for five minutes.

Identifying simple habits that you committed yourself to changing opens the doorway to important resources that *already exist within you*. These same internal resources are essential in changing your relationship with addiction. Of course, changing these practical and mundane habits are much easier to change than addictive processes tend to be. We obviously are not comparing apples with apples here; although some minor habits may be driven by underlying anxieties and worry, genuine addictive processes are much more complex. By and large, the emotional waters that run beneath addiction run deep. So, we need to start in the shallow end of the pool.

Unlike the simple habits that you have successfully overcome, addiction requires attending to something deeper, something more challenging. The practical skills you just identified are great resources to use to change your relationship to addiction. However, they are not sufficient on their own. To find the way through addiction we must find our way to its origins. What has addiction been attempting to self-medicate in the first place?

The Cues of Addiction

Taking a moment to reflect and begin *noticing when you use* offers the clearest pathway to identifying cues that set off addiction in your life. Exactly what is going on in these moments? There may be multiple cues occurring at any given time that could set your addictive process in motion.

Here is an example: In the thick of exam week, Miguel spotted his ex-girlfriend with a new partner. Although he had initiated the breakup, and it was quite amicable, the stress of exams combined with a surprising sense of loss was overwhelming him. To his credit, he hadn't used in months. Even though he had been through much worse over the past year, he had maintained a solid recovery through those tough times.

But there was something different this time... Without being aware of it, the combined recent events threw Miguel into the pain, loss, and devastation of his parents' contentious divorce. It happened so long ago that he rarely thought about it. But now it drew him into an emotional undertow he couldn't make sense of—after all, the specific events themselves weren't really all that difficult for him. Yet his current distress was disproportionate to what was happening in his life. Without awareness of so much unfinished business from long ago, Miguel became swept away in pain that he was unable to identify. His recovery had been solid for close to one year. But being unable to get a handle on what was occurring inside of him, Miguel began using pills again to quiet the pain.

A perfect storm blew into Miguel's life. What happened? Have you ever heard the phrase "under enough stress, we all regress"? Well, the emotional familiarity of loss during a very heightened time of stress had the power to unlock Miguel's compartmentalized hurt and pain from his childhood. The surge of emotion was so strong that, before he knew it, he was using.

The specifics of Miguel's story may be different from your own, but we all have been susceptible to the impact of the perfect storms in our lives. They have often led to falling off the wagon from our recovery.

Identifying Your Addiction Cues

This list is far from exhaustive, and you may add some examples from your own life.

Discrete events: Powerful specific events that shook you up or profoundly impacted you either in the past or recently, such as an enormous loss or an awful experience. These provide predictable cues for self-medicating with addiction.

Troubling childhood home or family or caregiving environment: Was growing up at home during your formative years painful or traumatizing? What was (or is) the vibe at home? Experiencing the impact of pain and negativity in our most important relationships is one of the most potent negative cues for using.

Current ongoing circumstances and environments: Are your work, school, or community environments or circumstances toxic, depleting, or demoralizing? When you leave work do you feel disrespected, overlooked, treated poorly? Does your significant-other relationship create harm or distress? Is school somewhere that leaves you feeling isolated or down on yourself? Having to spend large portions of each day in these environments can create a lot of emotional pain and erode your sense of self. This is very fertile ground to cue your addiction.

Disparaging social situations: Are your social groups toxic and triggering to your well-being? Do you feel devalued, ostracized, judged, invisible, or put down? Our social worlds create the fabric of our lives. Feeling alone, isolated, and less than can readily cue addiction as a quick and easy way to numb the pain.

Painful emotions from within: Many of us have an inner, felt-sense baseline of feeling less than, frightened, ashamed, unimportant, and powerless. These baseline feelings can have a profound effect on our relationship to addiction, and very consistently provide an ongoing cue for us to use.

Not being true to your core values: We have a genuine sense of what feels right and what feels wrong in the way that we approach and live our lives. Although these values and beliefs may remain unspoken, we usually have a clear sense of when we are living in harmony with them and when we have let ourselves down. This perceived personal failure can be a potent addiction activation cue.

Negative cultural elements and community influences: Many of us walk into places and spaces within our everyday lives concerned about safety as our first thought. Not everyone is free from worrying about feeling othered, marginalized, or worse. These fears, worries, and concerns are very present and real for so many of us. The constant impact of these realities is also a predictable cue for addiction.

The Power of Inner Narratives

In addition to emotion providing us with a finely tuned built-in alarm system capable of sending us lightning-quick safety signals in a moment's notice, it also provides us with the sophisticated ability to make meaning of situations as they occur. Similar to an enormous hard drive, our brain collects and retains data from everything that we have been exposed to and everything that we have learned throughout our entire lives. It uses this information to compare current situations to previous life experiences, so that we can take the most life-giving and danger-avoiding action possible in any given moment.

Once a cue triggers us, our brain instantaneously identifies similar experiences, and applies stored meaning to what is occurring. The stored meanings constitute our inner narratives. This process occurs rapidly and often outside of our conscious awareness. This information dictates whether we need to approach the situation or avoid it. We all experience objective situations in subjectively unique ways. It is the *meaning* that differs. Becoming aware of these stories is a crucial part of transforming your relationship with addictive behaviors. It is through understanding the personal meaning of our narratives that we can accurately interpret the cues and respond to them thoughtfully without moving immediately toward addiction.

And here is a key point: *It is not the cue in and of itself that sets addiction in motion; it's the uniquely personal meaning of the cue and the emotional feelings they stir up that are at the heart.* Identifying our inner narrative empowers us to target the parts of ourselves that have been beckoning for support and healing. Once we understand the meaning of our inner narratives clearly, we can replace our need for addiction with healthy methods for reassurance and peace.

Tolerating the Fire of Emotion

It is important to acknowledge that, as you courageously explore your inner world, it is predictable to feel emotionally flooded. That is not the intention of this work. However, it's a genuine possibility that merits mentioning.

Before going any further, it is important to locate where you are on the continuum of tolerating emotional experience. A side effect of addictive behavior is that it effectively turns down the dimmer switch of emotional awareness as a protective barrier from the overwhelm of facing our pain alone. The earlier in life we had to turn it down, the less emotionally fluent we became. The less experience we've had with our emotional worlds, the more intolerable the heat will be when we approach the burning buildings of our past.

Chronic addictive processes prevent us from facing life on life's terms. They block us from directly facing the challenges that come our way and from learning how to successfully navigate them. Although it may appear easier to avoid feeling overwhelmed or frightened, avoidance robs us of two crucial abilities: learning how to persevere in the face of life's challenges and experiencing success.

Avoidance keeps us stuck within false, life-depleting narratives. The more we avoid, the more it gives credence to our fears. Our fears reinforce old, uncontested narratives. These narratives give off more fear. More fear means we are more likely to use. This cycle prevents growth. We miss out on engaging with challenges that offer us opportunities to find solutions and, ultimately, the ability to trust ourselves.

ACTIVITY
The Window of Tolerance

The *window of tolerance* is a gauge to help you to better understand your ability to remain present, open, and responsive when you encounter challenging emotions and life experiences. This information is designed to help you develop the ability to remain in the middle "window" (between overactivated and shut down) as often as possible for optimal functioning and emotional balance. Shame and fear are the two most destabilizing emotions: They hold the potential to knock us out of our window of tolerance. When we fall outside of our window of tolerance, we shut down or get flooded with emotion and cannot process or navigate the situations we face.

Expanding your window of tolerance strengthens your ability to engage with emotion, accurately process what is occurring, and respond effectively in the moment. Tipping into *hyperarousal* emotionally floods our limbic system, rendering us unable to clearly analyze and process what is happening. It overwhelms our circuitry, depriving us of meaning from the challenges we encounter.

Conversely, when we tip into *hypoarousal*, our cortex overrides our emotions, and at best we go into our heads, or worse we dissociate and don't allow ourselves to feel. *Hypoarousal* insulates us from events and experiences that are occurring. It cuts us off from life, shuts us down, and robs us of experiencing anything. Shame is one of the most formidable culprits for tipping us outside of our window of tolerance, and tipping outside of our window is extremely fertile ground for using.

You may notice that whether your tendency is to hyperactivate or to deactivate; both provide perfect ingredients for the recipe of addiction. When we lose our emotional balance and equilibrium, the way in which we interact with other people tends to create disconnection. Given that these moments occur when we are emotionally flooded, we lose the option of reaching out for support and leaning into the people closest to us when we need them the most. That is extremely problematic when it comes to shame. Shame requires bringing the darkness of pain into the light of the people who care about us.

Pay attention as often as possible to your emotional state throughout the day. Become more acquainted with your inner terrain. The more aware you become of your emotional experience, the less frequently your emotions will ambush you and knock you out of your window of tolerance. There is a huge difference between you having your emotions, and your emotions having you. This is a powerful tool for keeping you on the path to transform your relationship with addiction.

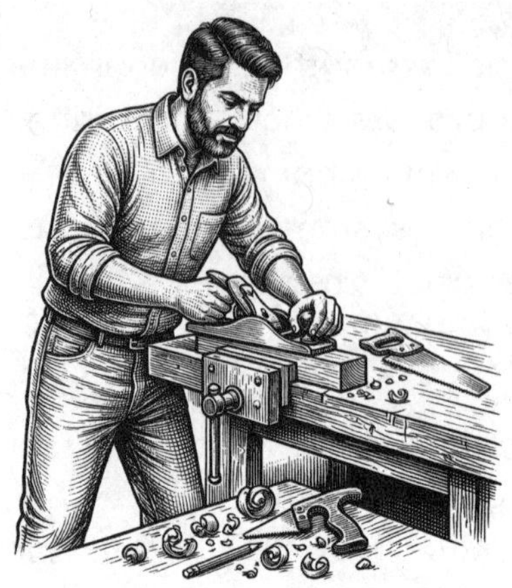

Dr. Rich's Impulse Remedy: Build Something

If you're itching to do something you might later regret, try channeling that energy into something productive. Make a birdhouse, a tree house, or a doghouse. Hell, just nail some pieces of wood together. I don't care what you make, just make something and let that urge pass on by.

Want more manly tips on Impulsive Behavior and Addiction? Explore the Gentlemental Health card on **ManTherapy.org.**

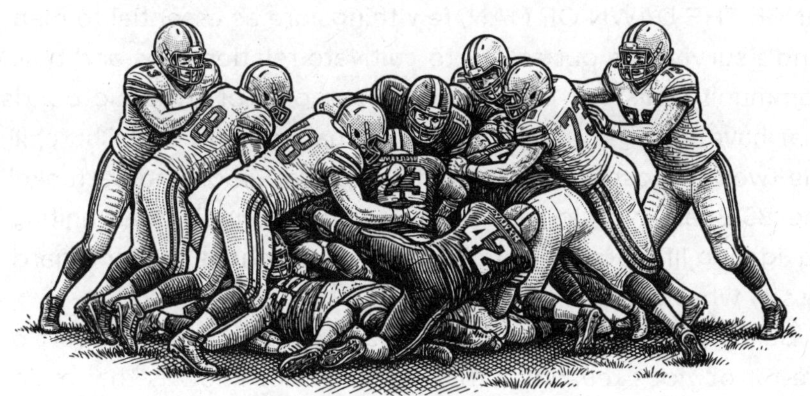

CHAPTER 7

RELATIONSHIPS AND FRIENDSHIPS

BUILDING RELATIONSHIPS IS A CONTACT SPORT

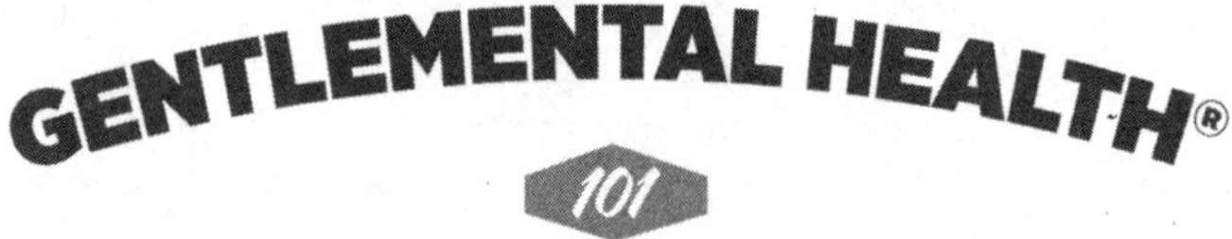

SINCE THE DAWN OF MAN, few things are as essential to mankind's survival as our ability to cultivate relationships and build community. History is filled with examples of dynamic bonds that have changed the course of humanity: FDR and Churchill, the Twelve Apostles, Antony and Cleopatra, Simon and Garfunkel, the '85 Bears. Nothing is more powerful than individuals uniting, navigating life together, and being in each other's corner regardless of what comes their way.

Building and maintaining relationships is an essential part of life for obvious reasons. What you may not know is that maintaining healthy relationships also has positive mental and physical health benefits. These include:

- Increased longevity

- Decreased risk of heart disease, stroke, dementia, diabetes, and high blood pressure

- Building a "psychological immune system" that buffers against stress, anxiety, and depression

- Boosted mood

- Improved coping skills and overall functioning

Healthy relationships also increase resilience and self-esteem, meaning you can bounce back quicker when life kicks you in the codpiece.

The unfortunate truth is that many men live in pursuit of rugged individualism and slip into lives of quiet desperation. Those who think that they're lone wolves are really just alone wolves. The root of this problem is that we often buy into our own BS when it comes to relationships. We believe that needing connection with a spouse, partner, friends, or loved ones makes us weak, that we should be able to nut up and get through life alone, or that good relationships should be easy.

Not only are those thoughts a load of hogwash, but they are also antithetical to what it means to be a human being, and they cut us off from one of the richest and most important aspects of life. Building and maintaining relationships, whether romantic or platonic, strikes directly at the core of what it means to be a man; to learn from the world around us, work at something meaningful, and strengthen ourselves and our communities. In short, being a man means using our effort and energy to make a positive impact.

Whether you're looking for ways to be a better husband, partner, or friend, there are plenty of strategies to help you navigate the world of connection and show up better for those you care about. To learn more about the importance of maintaining relationships and strategies for building them, let's check in with a qualified Man Therapist, Stan Tatkin.

BUILDING AND MAINTAINING RELATIONSHIPS

STAN TATKIN, PHD

Alongside our modern emphasis on autonomy, we see increasing evidence of loneliness inside and outside of marriages; a rising incidence of violence and alienation; and divorce rates that, while they may be decreasing, remain well above ideal.

Couples in distress too often turn to solutions like "You do your thing and I'll do my thing" or "You take care of yourself and I'll take care of myself." We hear pop psychology pronouncements such as "I'm not ready to be in a relationship" and "You have to love yourself before anyone can love you."

Is any of this true? Is it really possible to love yourself before someone ever loves you?

Think about it. How could this be true? If it were true, babies would come into this world already self-loving or self-hating. We know they don't. In fact, human beings don't start by thinking anything about themselves, good or bad. We learn to love ourselves precisely because we have experienced being loved by someone. We learn to take care of ourselves because somebody has taken care of us. Our self-worth and self-esteem also develop because of other people.

From the psychobiological perspective—and more specifically according to the insights of attachment theory—the bottom line is that most people need to feel closeness and ongoing connection with another human being. That is how we're hardwired. Yes, we need people, and in particular, we tend to need one special person who can provide a sense of safety and security in the world. That in turn can reduce day-to-day stress, increase self-confidence, and make it easier to venture out and slay all the dragons in the wider environment.

Some of us regard ourselves as basically "do-it-myself" people. I'm here to make the case that, really, none of us are. And in modern adult life, another person can greatly enrich your life and help you in whatever ways you may fall short if left to go it alone.

Here are a few practical examples:

- Another person can accurately guess, understand, and reflect back to you what you're going through.

- Another person can amplify your positive feelings and experiences, and assuage negative feelings and experiences.

- Another person can play with and (if needed) heal the baby within you.

- Another person can provide guidance about what to say or do when you're feeling lost or uncertain.

- Another person can step in and help when you're in trouble, emotionally or otherwise.

- Another person can boost your self-esteem when everything around you threatens to collapse.

- Another person can push you to be better than you ordinarily would be on your own.

- Another person can scratch the itch in that unreachable spot on your back (or in your soul).

People need people. And people have been in a lot of pain. Not simply due to the pandemic, which still reverberates for most folks. Increasing reliance on social media has taken its toll both socially and politically, leading to splits among couples, families, and friends. People are increasingly preoccupied with existential fears of climate change and have worries over the loss of liberal democracies both in the United States and abroad, as well as concerns about wars and growing division and tension among superpowers, a proliferation of guns and gun violence, the rise of antisemitism and racism, and growing tribalism. People are angsty, fearful, and some, increasingly aggressive and angry. In this post-pandemic stage, many show signs of PTSD among myriad other mental health issues.

These massive cultural issues affect our most intimate relationships, the context of our daily lives, and interactions with one another. Therefore, the need for secure functioning at home has increased. The home I speak of isn't a physical place. It's our closest relationships, starting with our partners, and then our children, then other family members, friends, and neighbors.

The truth is, humankind has always faced existential threats. Yes, the world is more complex today than it was when we were simply hunters and gatherers. Yet, we've evolved to this complexity—even created it. Our safety and security, our comfort, our only real solace in an unpredictable, indifferent, and often violent world is and always has been our relationship with loved ones.

We know, from more than one longitudinal study, that happiness, physical and mental health, and longevity hinges on having at least one secure-functioning relationship in our life (Bradt 2015). Just one. A secure-functioning relationship is an organic antidepressant, an organic anxiolytic (antianxiety), an organic psychostimulant, and an organic mood stabilizer. Not just any relationship yields these positive effects: most relationships are insecure functioning and have the opposite impact—increased unhappiness, increased interpersonal stress, increased threat perception and memory, shorter lifespan, plus wear and tear on cardiovascular, autoimmune, inflammatory, and metabolic systems.

Most everyone can achieve secure functioning if partners decide that is how they wish to run their partnership. And a secure-functioning partnership can provide a sorely needed source of solace amid all kinds of challenges and threats from an ever-changing world.

As humans, we need this.

Think of secure functioning as a culture—one that is cocreated and continuously shaped by both of you. Imagine you are with others who form the culture you're cocreating, with a block of clay between you. Together, you are the creators, molding and shaping the clay to your liking. This living piece of art represents meaning, purpose, vision, culture, ethics, values, dreams, goals, aspirations, and behavioral restrictions that will protect you from harming the other, whether purposely or inadvertently.

Alternatively, you might imagine yourselves as architects, designing the home that is your relationship. Are you predicting and planning for the long run? Are you considering what could go wrong? Are you thinking long and hard about its structure, organization, and sturdiness in case of earthquakes, bad weather, fires, and such? Freedom must be contained in an agreed upon structure; otherwise, freedom could become confinement or chaos.

As a couple, a two-person psychological system, you must acknowledge your separateness and at the same time recognize your interdependence. As a team or alliance, everything you do affects the other—positively or negatively. Cause and effect are constant reminders that your fates are bound to each other. No good or bad act by one won't be returned in some way and at some point. This is a team sport, not a solo one—unless the two of you agree to play it that way. If so, be very clear what that means and how it will work both now and in the future.

Secure-functioning adult relationships, whether you are married, partnered, intimate sexually or not, must be fully informed and consensual, mutually designed, and based on terms and conditions that each person deems fair, just, and mutually sensitive. People are free to make any arrangements, agreements, or lifestyle choices so long as they agree and know precisely what they are agreeing to. Being able to do this depends on being interdependent, rather than codependent.

Putting Yourself Out There

Many people are excited about dating, but have become overwhelmed and feel defeated. Some are ready to call it quits. Others are just setting themselves up for future failure. What these individuals have in common is that they are unclear about why they want to date, the kind of person they want to date, and the kind of relationship they wish to end up in.

The topics I'll cover here are all ideally ones to think about before you begin dating, to help you gear up for the process. However, even if you are actively dating, it's not too late to go back to basics and resolve any issues and concerns you still have. Or if you've come to a point of feeling your years of effort have been in vain, then please don't despair: there is hope!

People have many reasons for dating: they may want to get married, start a family, avoid being alone, establish independence, expand their circle of friends, or seek new experiences. All these are valid reasons, but here I'm going to assume you want to date because you are serious about finding a committed partner. In that case, it's helpful to start by examining the ideas and preconceptions you have about the kind of partner, and kind of relationship, you want. Your ideas are what you bring to the table, and as such they play a role in determining where and with whom you end up.

I'm going to venture out on a limb by saying this: the chances are pretty good—whether you admit it or not—that you are looking for one special person, not two or three or more. Chances are also pretty good that you are seeking both some degree of relationship permanence and some degree of interdependency. At the same time, I would hazard a guess that you are wondering if this kind of committed relationship is possible for you. Even if you want to believe it is possible, you may wonder if it is really worth pursuing. Maybe you feel you're not "made" for relationships. Or you think pairing up is a trap you'd be smart to avoid. In short, you may be experiencing a big dose of dating-and-relationship skepticism right about now.

There is a reason that seeking a partner isn't as straightforward as, say, going through the process of buying a new car or new house. When it comes to courtship, biological and social influences can be at odds. It may be that your biological hard wiring leads you to want a committed relationship, but that the prevailing mores in your social group carry a strong pull in the opposing direction. For instance, if you're a young person and your friends spend more time socializing in groups than dating, you are likely to do the same, regardless of other inclinations you may feel. Similarly, if you watch movies or TV shows in which multiple partners, or many partners in quick succession, are the norm, that may have an impact on your choices. These kinds of social trends can cast doubt on what you otherwise would consider the best way to form relationships.

Before we go any further, I want to talk about some common ideas—I would call them myths—about love relationships. Many ideas that I believe make it harder to find a partner—or at least to have a happy experience doing so—have taken hold to varying degrees in our collective minds. If you are interested in understanding how you are wired for dating, and want to use that understanding to your best advantage, I suggest carefully reassessing each of these myths.

MYTH 1: LOVE IS ALL YOU NEED TO MAKE A RELATIONSHIP SUCCEED

Perhaps when you think about "love," you're hoping for a giddy, mushy, thunderstruck feeling, the promise of which lures you into the dating journey (and that later entices you to make promises you otherwise never would). If this is the case, I have to say no: that sort of love is not all you need. For starters, along with that mushy feeling, a variety of other ingredients are essential if a dating relationship is going to lead to a long-term love relationship. Above all else, you and your partner need to offer each other safety and security. You need to be able to protect each other and count on each other, and find a way of being together that is mutually beneficial, fair, just, and sensitive. This is not the heart-racing thrill of love, but it is the stuff of lasting relationship. Love matters, of course, but it has to be demythologized before you can venture to live according to any maxim that uses the word. One way you can bust any myths you have about love is to carefully consider what love means to you.

MYTH 2: YOU HAVE TO LOVE YOURSELF BEFORE YOU CAN LOVE SOMEONE ELSE

If this were true, a baby would have to love itself before it was able to love its mother. But that's not what happens: a baby learns to love from being loved. For a baby, there is no loving without feeling loved, or vice versa. The two work in tandem, inseparable. In fact, the baby experiences being loved and loving before it has any concept of what love is. Moreover, self-love becomes meaningful only after a child experiences a sense of separate self. That typically occurs after a child's first birthday. (Pediatrician T. Berry Brazelton and others have researched and written at length on this topic.) Suffice it to say that, in our earliest stages of development, love is like a vast ocean whose waves do not distinguish between self and other. You learn to love by engaging with others, period. It can't be done alone.

MYTH 3: YOU HAVE TO LEARN TO TAKE CARE OF YOURSELF BEFORE YOU CAN START DATING

Myth #3 is related to Myth #2. People who espouse this myth may be fearful of becoming too dependent on another person. They may lack confidence in their ability to leave a romantic relationship when and if necessary. Fear of abandonment eclipses all other matters, including their own happiness in a relationship. The notion that you have to take care of yourself first risks presupposing that you and your partner couldn't share the kind of mutuality in which you both agree to take care of each other; or it suggests that you do not trust and welcome that mutual responsibility.

MYTH 4: YOU SHOULDN'T RELY ON ONLY ONE PERSON FOR YOUR WELL-BEING

In other words, no potential partner will be able to satisfy all your wants and needs; Myth #4 is in that sense a permutation of Myth #3. And in fact, there is some actual truth to this truism. It is never healthy to restrict your relational needs to one person, to the exclusion of all others. Couples who isolate themselves in this way, without a social network, are at risk of falling into what is known as a folie à deux. But this is not what I mean when I cite this idea as a "myth." I do so because many people use it to define a pro-self rather than pro-relationship stance, and to avoid creating greater closeness with a partner. You can and should be able to depend on just one person—namely, the person you choose—as long as that person is dependable and you, too, are dependable. Believing that relying on one person is a bad idea prevents you from dating someone with whom you will be able to create a relationship that offers the safety and security you need.

MYTH 5: I NEED TO FIND MY SOUL MATE

You might feel that you are a romantic and that destiny dictates you find the one person who can make you happy. I'm afraid that sort of happiness will elude you; again, it's a numbers problem. Moreover, you change as you age. What you think will make you happy now may not be what you want or need five, ten, or twenty years from now. Some people pattern their ideal partner after their continuously changing feeling state. A real person could never compete with that. For both these reasons—the numbers, and the changeability of human nature—rather than holding out for the one and only perfect person out there, I suggest you think in terms of many possible people, any of whom could love and accept you as you change and grow throughout your lifetime. Your brain picks partners based on familiarity, not on the possibility you shared a previous life or anything of that nature. In truth, there are many, many, many potential soul mates for you out there. And all are unique. Every primary love relationship is unique, like a fingerprint, and cannot be duplicated.

Could many potential partners be your soul mates? Only you can answer that question—or, more accurately, your brain can. Your subconscious mind will consider anyone with whom you feel familiarity and recognition a good candidate—at least in the short run. Then it will be up to you to go through the dating process and decide if that other person is a viable long-term prospect. As far as soul mate status, I leave it to you and your eventual partner to decide whether you want to give each other that title.

MYTH 6: DATING IS FOR THE YOUNG—I'M TOO OLD

No ambiguity about this one: it's not true at all. Generally speaking, as we age, we become more fluid and flexible with ourselves and others. We are more aware of our mortality and of the fact that we can't do everything. We have a better sense of what we do and don't like, and our priorities are different—perhaps relationships and family have become more important than career. When it comes time to meet a new partner, we can present ourselves in a more realistic fashion. Of course, some dating disadvantages can also come with age. For example, if you have loved and lost, you may be reluctant to try again. And even though you have the natural confidence that comes with age, it may elude you in the dating arena due to age-related image concerns.

Romantic Partnership and Navigating Relationship Conflict

When I see partners in a successfully maintained couple bubble, one standout feature is their ability to care for, influence, and manage one another, much the way expert parents do with their children. Both partners seem to have read and carefully studied the owner's manual for their relationship and for each other. Each is familiar with operational details that no one outside of the bubble is likely to know.

For instance, these partners know what has the most power to push the other's buttons. When the other is feeling bad, they immediately sense why. Not only that, they know how to remedy the situation. They know the right words to say, or deeds to perform, that have the power to elevate, relieve, excite, soothe, or heal each other. From a neuroscience perspective, these partners possess well-functioning prefrontal cortices; well-balanced left and right brains; well-developed smart vagal systems; well-regulated breath and vocal control; and honed communication skills that keep love close and war at a far distance.

How did they get to be so adept? Are such people perhaps in possession of a perfect partner gene? Trust me, no. Do they have some kind of secret superpower that allows them to manage their partner emotionally? Well, maybe. As I said earlier, some of us got a better start in life than others, with lots of positive interactions with safe adults who were interested in and curious about us. We all come to the table with primitive parts of our brain that don't want us to be harmed and ambassadors that can be annoying. Truth is, we can be, all of us, pains in the rear. When we recite our relationship vows, perhaps we should say, "I take you as my pain in the rear, with all your history and baggage, and I take responsibility for all prior injustices you endured at the hands of those I never knew because you now are in my care."

Hmm. How many people would be willing to say those vows? And yet, in my practice and research, that is exactly what I see couples in secure relationships doing. It is a conscious choice they make. They agree to take each other on "as is" and take responsibility for one another's care. As experts who understand their partner, they do what's necessary to relieve the other's distress or to amplify their elation. To many partners who find themselves at the mercy of each other's moods, this kind of expertise may indeed seem like a secret superpower they'd do almost anything to obtain.

The role of the primary partner is a big one: it entails taking good care of another human pain in the rear. The only way for this to work is for both partners to become experts on one another. With this kind of arrangement, nobody really loses and everybody truly wins. You can think of it as a kind of pay-to-play version of romance. It is, make no mistake, an investment in your future.

THE TWO OR THREE THINGS THAT MAKE YOUR PARTNER FEEL GOOD

How many people actually know how to spontaneously make their partner feel happy and loved? I'm talking here of a phrase, a deed, or an expression aimed at one's partner meant specifically to uplift them. I have seen partners married for thirty years who appear dumbfounded when challenged to brighten, move, charm, or otherwise enamor one another. Yet, this ability to spontaneously and predictably shift or elevate your partner's mood or emotional state is a crucial aspect of being an expert on your partner.

In my work with couples, I have found most people don't want their partner to change, not really. They fundamentally appreciate their partners as they are. But what people do want is to know how to influence, motivate, and otherwise have a positive effect on their partner. They want to avoid pushing the other's buttons. But that's not enough. They also want to know the antidotes to apply when things go awry. They want to be privy to when and where their partner has an itch so they can scratch it for them.

In this way, couples seek to become competent managers of each other. In fact, their competence as partners is not unlike the competence of parents who want to soothe their child's painful feelings and cultivate positive ones. It also can be compared to the role of a regulator. Partners who are competent managers help regulate each other's moods and energy levels. As regulators, each continually monitors the other and knows when to jump in and throw a switch to help restore balance in the direction of those things that make the partner feel good.

More than just a safe environment, the couple bubble is a place for partners to feel excitement, enrichment, and most importantly, attraction. I'm not speaking here about physical attraction; I mean the kind of attraction that serves as glue to hold the relationship together. Unfortunately, fear is often the glue holding couples together. Fear may be useful for keeping a partner in line, but it obviously is counter to the notion of a couple bubble. We should want to be in the bubble; we shouldn't feel we have to be there. We want to be with our partner because there is no other place in the world we'd rather be. Our attraction is based on what we do for one another that no one else can or wants to do. Couples who don't use this kind of attraction as their glue are doomed to fail sooner or later.

ACTIVITY
What Can Uplift Your Partner?

Are you aware of what things you can say or do that have the power to relieve distress and uplift your partner? Take a minute and think about these now.

You may find it helpful to begin with the list of vulnerabilities. For each of the two or three things that make your partner feel bad, you probably can identify something that will mollify the bad feeling. For instance, if my history has me doubting my worth as a parent, my partner can predictably brighten my mood with a spontaneous "You're such a good father," delivered right into my eyes.

Check the list you come up with against the antidotes, which might give you additional ideas.

You may also want to create a list of the things your partner can (and does) do that please and uplift you. If you are doing this exercise together, you can create separate lists for each other and then compare notes.

ACTIVITY
The Emote Me Game

You can play this game with your partner, each taking turns to "emote" the other. Or you can practice it without telling your partner what you're doing. Either way, you stand to learn a lot about your relationship.

1. Say or do something to make your partner smile brightly. Drawing upon your knowledge of your partner, try to anticipate what will bring a smile to their face, then watch and see if it works. For example, you might give your partner a back rub or relate a special shared memory.

2. Now say something complimentary about your partner that will profoundly move them. You will know you have succeeded if you bring tears to your partner's eyes. I don't mean tears of sadness, but the moistness that comes when we feel deeply touched. Brief, declarative statements are most likely to succeed. Long, drawn-out statements will fail. Avoid adding qualifications. For example, your partner may be moved if you say, "You're the most trustworthy person I know," but saying "You're a very trustworthy person...most of the time" is unlikely to produce the desired effect. Neither will a lazy compliment, such as "You know how much I like your cooking." That isn't very moving if you're just repeating what you think your partner already knows. And don't always expect immediate results. If your partner doesn't respond to a compliment, take that as information about what affects them, and try something else.

3. Finally, say or do something that causes your partner to get excited. You can see excitement in the eyes: they widen and the pupils dilate, if only for an instant. Your partner's

face may become redder and their vocal tone may become higher in pitch and louder.

4. If you are playing this game together, don't ask your partner what will work. It's your job as the expert to find this out. Don't ask your partner if what you said or did worked either. Look for the clues; notice your partner's reaction. Through this process, you both build your expertise. You will both receive benefits. Remember, you are wired together!

5. The two of you can play the Emote Me game whenever you feel like it. Experiment with different positive effects: make your partner relax, make your partner laugh, or anything else you can think of.

The principle here is that partners who are experts on one another know how to please and soothe each other. This means becoming familiar with your partner's primary vulnerabilities and knowing the antidotes that are effective for each.

ACTIVITY
Wave the Flag of Friendliness

One of the best ways partners can avoid war, especially when distress is mounting, is to quickly wave the flag of friendliness. You can do it. Your partner can do it. It doesn't really matter; all it takes is one person to make the first move.

The smart vagus nerve is one of the most important ambassadors when it comes to avoiding war. The smart vagus not only allows us to take a deep breath before acting but also helps us modulate our voice to signal friendliness through tone and volume.

Our other ambassadors, particularly the orbitofrontal cortex—which allows us to step into someone else's shoes—can calm down our amygdalae before they scream red alert over what is actually a nonexistent threat. Make it clear you understand where your partner is coming from and open the door to a friendly discussion about your respective points of view. Using a familiar term of endearment shows that your love hasn't been lost in the scuffle. Yet other ambassadors specialize in helping us produce facial expressions that can ease our partner's distress. An unequivocal smile can communicate goodwill more rapidly than any words.

Sound silly? I don't think so. You can try this technique at any point, though it may not always be effective during a heated dispute. Nevertheless, many a war has been avoided with a friendly smile, a well-placed touch, and a reassuring voice.

IT'S ALL JUST BLAH-BLAH-BLAH

When you wave the flag of friendliness, you in essence take a shortcut. You circumvent all the angry words that make up a fight, and instead communicate with a single gesture. The same can hold true during a fight. Sometimes when you have reached an apparent impasse, the most effective thing you or your partner can do is just...shut up.

I mean that literally. Stop speaking. Recognize that you are threatened and nothing of interpersonal value can come out of your mouth until your chill is back online.

Our left brain is wired to be highly verbal and logical. It specializes in processing detailed information and readily engages with all the minutiae that go into an argument. At its best, it can sort out the minutiae and settle the argument; at its worst—directed by the amygdalae—it produces a lot of blah-blah-blah. What comes out of threatened partners' mouths is garbage, useless blather whose only purpose is to fend off attack or aggression. It's as if both brains are interacting amygdalae to amygdalae, with no evidence of flexibility, complexity, creativity, or contingency. What you say in this situation will only need to be discounted later, when you and your partner attempt to deal with all the hurtful things your amygdalae did to one another.

So, what I'm suggesting is that you shift your partner toward friendliness and away from threat. If you can do this, you will have aborted a fight.

Bro Code: Building Better Friendships with Your Dudes

First and foremost, it is important to understand the one basic and counterintuitive foundation that will aid in preserving and enhancing your male friendships: a healthy and steady primary relationship with a spouse or partner, if you have one. If you don't have one of these, that's ok—a good and old friend can be a great model. The point is that secure attachment is like a magnet that attracts more secure attachment. Maintaining healthy relationship with your buddies is best modeled and practiced at home with your main, #1 person because the same rules apply: honest and vulnerable communication, commitment to quality time together, and knowing someone deeply enough to become their go-to.

One of the things I see with people who have known each other a long time is "We're beyond all that now." This is a common notion, and I believe it is a mistake. Even when you've been bros for a while, I believe you should remain in teenager mode, at least to some degree. It's the teenager mode—the same one you both were likely in when you met your best male friends—that helps create novelty, excitement, and the desirable kind of strangeness.

My teenager mode experiences are mostly related to travel, especially since I founded the PACT Institute to train therapists. I travel constantly to training sites, both around the country and internationally, and love seeing new sights and meeting new people, sometimes bringing my friends along. Traveling, for us, is a team process. We have traveling down to a science. One thing we have learned is to pack using carry-ons only, even when going to faraway places for long periods. My friends and I make sure to share leadership roles. One is "Scout," who studies ahead and plans; and I'm "Tracker," who is scanning for spontaneity and fun. We meet folks on planes and trains, and often in the strangest of places. It seems that wherever we go, something unexpected happens, from the sublime to the ridiculous. But the more crucial part, beyond the pleasure of each other's company, is the respect that we have for one another's strengths and how we design things to do that amplify them.

I'm not suggesting that you need to travel in order to keep your friendship fresh. Anything you do that is novel or adventuresome can put you back in teenager mode. Part of all of us crave newness, and a surefire way to experience that newness is by scheduling and bringing each other into novel adventures. Push each other to do things that you otherwise might not do. Often this includes the art of negotiation. For example, one evening my friend wanted to have a drink at our favorite haunt, and I wanted to see a movie. You would only have needed the most basic sherlocking skills to recognize that I'm not a fan of going out just for drinks, and to discover that my friend prefers activities that allow us to give each other more attention. So what did we do? We ended up going to the movie first, and having a drink afterward to talk about the movie. We both won, and also both did something we didn't like. I'm sharing a bit of my own experience to illustrate some of the ways in which a friendship is always an adventure, always in development. I don't care how "beyond all that" you think you are; friends can and will get on each other's nerves. They fight about stupid stuff. They say things they wish they hadn't said. They have bad days. But that shouldn't scare you from committing to your homies.

Dr. Rich's Relationship Remedy: Bowling

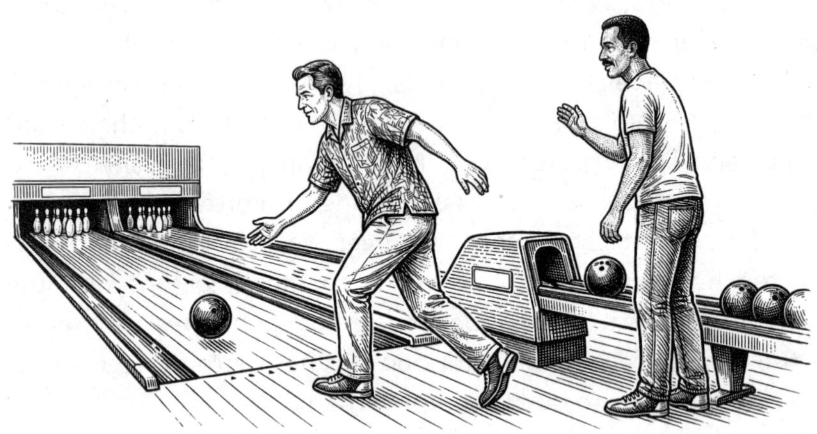

For thousands, maybe even millions, of years, men have gathered together to relax. Sometimes at the foot of finely polished lanes. So, grab your ball, give her a nice shine, and get out there. The relationship-boosting benefits of striking pins down with friends are endless.

Want more manly tips on Relationships and Friendships? Explore the Gentlemental Health card on **ManTherapy.org**.

ONWARD AND UPWARD

TAKING CARE OF YOUR MENTAL HEALTH IS THE MANLIEST THING YOU CAN DO

There is no way to happiness, happiness is the way.
  —Thich Nhat Hanh

Well, that was a lot of information to take in. Sometimes books are just so many words! My hope is that you can keep this guide within reach when you find yourself suddenly struggling with any of the subjects covered on these pages. Perhaps you'll find yourself reading a chapter down the road that gives you an insight, inspiration or nudge you need to make the right move. We certainly haven't covered everything related to men's mental health, but we hope you have found something interesting, useful or relevant to you.

No one gets through this world without facing challenges, setbacks and heartbreaks. That's just part of the deal with being human. And what's an even better part of being human is all the fun, joy, love, purpose, meaning, and happiness that is out there waiting for us.

There are some very essential questions that each of us needs to ponder and answer for ourselves: What are our priorities and what kind of a life do we want? How do we measure success? What fills our cup and helps us sleep well at night? What do we look forward to that gets us excited about getting out of bed? Who and what matters most in our lives? And what makes us happy? Here are just a few parting shots of advice as you move forward out there on the front lines of life:

1. Realize that no matter what you are facing, there is a way forward.

2. Take small steps and any action that will set a new direction.

3. Acknowledge you are a work in progress.

4. Be honest with yourself, be willing to do the work, and be willing to ask for help if you need it.

5. Take care of yourself (body, mind and spirit).

6. Recognize it's all connected, and every choice matters.

7. Make the people and things around you better.

8. Find meaning and purpose in your life.

9. Have fun, laugh, relax and smell the roses.

10. Spend more time with family and friends.

I'm reminded of a very simple but essentially important Buddhist philosophy about living for the moment: Today is the only day. It reminds us that there is really only one day. Yesterday is dead and over. Tomorrow is not yet born. Today is the only day that matters. Life is full of heartbreak and joy. We need to embrace each as we keep moving forward, controlling what we can, and doing our best to succeed, thrive and matter.

I hope you find joy and happiness more often than not.

—Joe Conrad

ACKNOWLEDGEMENTS

There are many people to thank that have played a role in developing Man Therapy and getting this book published. Thanks to Jarrod Hindman and Sally Spencer-Thomas (founder of the Carson J. Spencer Foundation), my original Man Therapy partners. The incredible teams at Cactus who created the campaign include my partner Norm Shearer and the OGs Elliott Nordstrom and Jorge Lamora. A big shout out to the Cactus creative teams over the years that have kept the campaign fresh and sharp. To the one and only John Arp, the actor who brought Dr. Rich Mahogany to life. Man Therapy would not have been possible without the generous support of the Anschutz Foundation and the Colorado Department of Public Health & Environment, Office of Suicide Prevention. A big thanks to our Man Therapy partners throughout the U.S. who are champions for the brand and are making men's mental health a priority in their community.

Many incredible partnerships and ripples have flowed out of Man Therapy, including the founding of Grit Digital Health in 2015 that brought together a team of talented and committed individuals who create mental health and well-being platforms for college students, veterans, first responders and the U.S. military. Thank you to the amazing team at Grit Digital Health who has worked to make the Man Therapy platform better and our network stronger, including Colin Tackett, Paige Beaufort, Trip Starkey, Thomas Vossler, Daniel Fong, Mikayla Smith, Frank Lahtinen, Doug Sparks, Nathaan Demers, and Andrew Baker. Tip of the cap to Trip Starkey for the great conversations about this project and for the significant writing and editing work you contributed to this book.

Today, Man Therapy is a men's mental health platform that continues its mission of helping men not only survive but thrive. Millions of men, and the people who love them, have visited the site, with more than 650,000 Head Inspections completed. A four-year clinical study sponsored by the CDC found that Man Therapy is an effective intervention that improves help-seeking behavior. This little campaign out of Colorado continues to make an impact with partners throughout the world. It has been an honor to be a part of this campaign.

Thank you to the wonderful team at New Harbinger Publications for being great partners, curating the content with your team of authors, and bringing this important subject to men and the women who love them. A special thank you to Glenn Schiraldi, Edmund Bourne, Randy Patterson, Matthew McKay, Peter Rogers, Michael Barnett, and Stan Tatkin for contributing your voice to this work and championing men's mental health.

And finally, to the primary source of purpose and meaning in my life, my wife Erin and our children Jordan, Mikayla and Jackson. You'll always be my North star.

REFERENCES

Alexander, B. K. 2008.*The Globalization of Addiction: A Study in Poverty of the Spirit*. Oxford: Oxford University Press.

Blanco, C., C. Lopez-Quintero, D. S. Hasin, J. P. de Los Cobos, A. Pines, S. Wang, and B. F. Grant. 2011. "Probability and Predictors of Remission from Lifetime Nicotine, Alcohol, Cannabis, or Co-caine Dependence: Results from the National Epidemiologic Survey on Alcohol and Related Conditions."*Society for the Study of Addiction* 106(3): 657–669.

Bradt, G. 2015. "The Secret of Happiness Revealed By Harvard Study." *Forbes*, May 27. https://www.forbes.com/sites/georgebradt/2015/05/27/the-secret-of-happiness-revealed-by-harvard-study.

Felitti, V. J. 2002. "The Relation Between Adverse Childhood Experiences and Adult Health: Turning Gold into Lead." *Permanente Journal* 6: 44–47.

Finberg, A., dir. 2015. *The Business of Recovery*. Los Angeles: Greg Horvath Productions; Distribber.

Follette, V. M., and J. Pistorello. 2007. *Finding Life Beyond Trauma: Using Acceptance and Commitment Therapy to Heal from Post-Traumatic Stress and Trauma-Related Problems*. Oakland, CA: New Harbinger Publications.

Fredrickson, B. L. 2009. *Positivity: Top-Notch Research Reveals the 3 to 1 Ratio That Will Change Your Life*. New York: Three Rivers Press.

Hasin, D. S., F. S. Stinson, E. Ogburn, and B. F. Grant. 2007. "Prevalence, Correlates, Disability, and Comorbidity of DSM Alcohol Abuse in the United States: Result from the National Epidemiological Survey on Alcohol and Related Conditions." *Archives of General Psychiatry* 64(7): 830–842.

Heyman, G. 2009. *Addiction: A Disorder of Choice.* Boston: Harvard University Press.

Kessler, R. C., K. A. McGonagle, S. Zhao, C. B. Nelson, M. Hughes, S. Eshleman, H. U. Wittchen, and K. S. Kender. 1994. "Lifetime and 12-Month Prevalence of DSM-III-R Psychiatric Disorders in the United States." *Archives of General Psychiatry* 51: 8–19.

Kessler, R. C., P. Berglund, O. Demler, R. Jin, K. R. Merikangas, and E. E. Walters. 2005. "Lifetime Prevalence and Age-of-Onset Distributions of DSM-IV Disorders in the National Comorbidity Survey Replication." *Archives of General Psychiatry* 62: 593–602.

Kirschman, E. 2004. *I Love a Fire Fighter: What the Family Needs to Know.* New York: Guilford Press.

Lyubomirsky, S. 2007. *The How of Happiness: A Scientific Approach to Getting the Life You Want.* New York: Penguin Books.

Maté, G. 2007. *In the Realm of Hungry Ghosts: Close Encounters with Addiction.* Berkeley: North Atlantic Books

Medoff, M. 1986. "In Praise of Teachers." *New York Times Magazine,* November 9. http://www.nytimes.com/2+9+/11/09/magazine/in-praise-of-teachers.html.

Prigerson, H. G., A. J. Bierhals, S. V. Kasl, C. F. Reynolds 3rd, M. K. Shear, N. Day, L. C. Beery, J. T. Newsom, and S. Jacobs. 1997. "Traumatic Grief as a Risk Factor for Mental and Physical Morbidity." *American Journal of Psychiatry,* 154: 616–623.

Werner, E. E. 1992. "The Children of Kauai: Resiliency and Recovery in Adolescence and Adulthood." *Journal of Adolescent Health,* 13: 262–268.

Wilson, Reid. 1996. *Don't Panic.* New York: HarperCollins.

Joe Conrad is a creative entrepreneur and digital health pioneer who believes that the power of innovation and technology can solve any problem. As the founder of Cactus, a full-service creative agency, and Grit Digital Health, a behavioral health technology company, Joe's work is committed to transcending barriers, driving behavior change, and helping individuals and organizations thrive. Joe and his team are the creators of Man Therapy®, an evidence-based platform and men's mental health brand. Joe lives in Colorado.

Contributor Matthew McKay, PhD, is a professor at the Wright Institute in Berkeley, CA. He is coauthor of The *Dialectical Behavior Therapy Skills Workbook*, *The Relaxation and Stress Reduction Workbook*, *Thoughts and Feelings*, *When Anger Hurts*, and others. His books combined have sold more than five million copies. He received his PhD in clinical psychology from the California School of Professional Psychology. In private practice, he specializes in the treatment of post-traumatic stress disorder (PTSD) and anxiety. He lives and works in the greater San Francisco Bay Area.

Contributor Stan Tatkin, PsyD, MFT, is a clinician, teacher, and developer of the Psychobiological Approach to Couple Therapy (PACT). He has a clinical practice in Calabasas, CA; where he has specialized for the last twenty years in working with couples and individuals who wish to be in relationships. He and his wife, Tracey Boldemann-Tatkin, developed the PACT Institute for the purpose of training other psychotherapists to use this method in their clinical work.

Contributor Edmund J. Bourne, PhD, has specialized in the treatment of anxiety, panic, phobias and other stress-related disorders for more than three decades. His self-help books have reached more than a million people and have been translated into numerous languages. Bourne currently resides in San Diego, CA. While partly retired, he speaks with telephone clients for brief therapy. For information, please visit his website **www. helpforanxiety.com**.

Contributor Glenn R. Schiraldi, PhD, has served on the stress management faculties at The Pentagon; the International Critical Incident Stress Foundation; and the University of Maryland, where he received the Outstanding Teaching Award in addition to other teaching and service awards. His books on stress-related topics have been translated into sixteen languages, and include: *The Resilience Workbook*; *The Self-Esteem Workbook*; *Ten Simple Solutions for Building Self-Esteem*; and *The Anger Management Sourcebook*. Glenn's writing has been recognized by various scholarly and popular sources, including *The Washington Post*, *American Journal of Health Promotion*, *Mind/Body Health Review*, and the *International Stress and Tension Control Society Newsletter*. Learn more at **www.resiliencefirst.com**.

Contributor Randy J. Paterson, PhD, is a psychologist, and author of *How to Be Miserable* and *How to Be Miserable in Your Twenties*. He is director of Changeways Clinic in Vancouver, BC, Canada; and provides training programs across Canada and internationally on evidence-based mental health practice. Learn more a**t www.randypaterson.com**.

Contributor Michael Barnett, LPCC, is a certified trainer in emotionally focused therapy (EFT) who has added to the canon of EFT training by helping clinicians work more effectively with trauma and addiction through the EFT lens. Barnett specializes in the use of EFT as a humanistic/experiential, attachment-based therapy to transform clients' relationship with their addictive processes. He is codirector of the Emotionally Focused Therapy Center of Los Angeles, and founder of the Atlanta Community for Emotionally Focused Therapy. He resides in La Crescenta, CA.

BOOKS *to* HELP YOU HEAL

Written by
Real Experts *for* Real Change

For more than fifty years, New Harbinger
has published practical, compassionate
books grounded in psychology, mindfulness,
and the science of behavior change.
Explore our full catalog of workbooks,
guides, and resources for every step
of your healing journey.

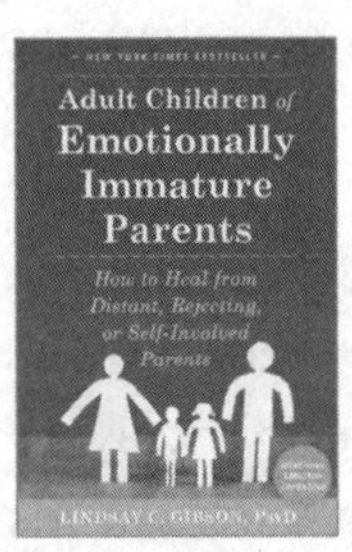

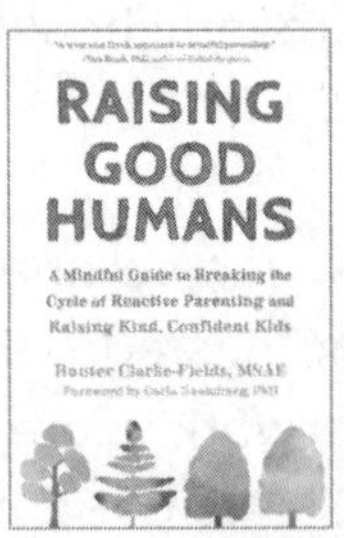

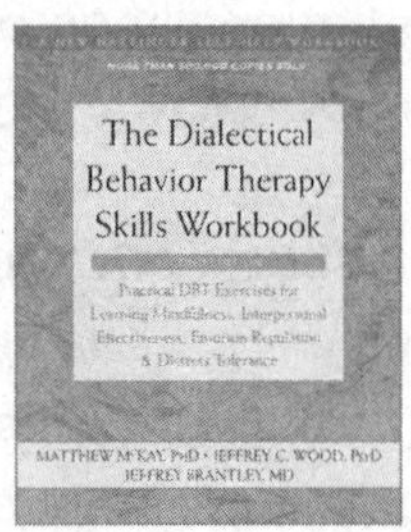

Discover more at **newharbinger.com**

new**harbinger**publications